Just Stay ...

JUST STAY ...
A Couple's Last Journey Together

JENNIFER FAZAKERLEY   HELEN BUTLIN -BATTLER   GRACE BRADISH

Words Indeed Publishing Inc.

TORONTO

Words Indeed Publishing Inc., Toronto, Canada
www.wordsindeed.ca

For more information please visit:
www.juststay.ca

ISBN: 978-0-9865166-5-8

Library and Archives Canada Cataloguing in Publication

Fazakerley, Jennifer, 1974-
Just stay— : a couple's last journey together / Jennifer Fazakerley,
Grace Bradish, Helen Buttlin-Battler.

ISBN 978-0-9865166-5-8

1. Fazakerley, Rob, d. 2010. 2. Pancreas—Cancer—Patients—
Biography. 3. Pancreas—Cancer—Patients—Home care.
4. Pancreas—Cancer—Patients—Family relationships. I. Bradish,
Grace, 1955- II. Buttlin-Battler, Helen, 1968- III. Title.

RC280.P25F39 2012   616.994'37092   C2012-905664-2

Cover: Val Cooke
Book design & typesetting: Anne Vellone
Photographs: Jennifer Fazakerley; front cover: Mark Spowart
Photo retouching: courtesy of Robert Wood, Clarity Colour
Copyediting: John Parry
Printing services: Advertek Printing

A portion of the proceeds of this book will be donated to cancer research.

Printed and bound in Canada on acid-free paper

If I accept death, then my tree greens,
since dying increases life.
If I plunge into the death encompassing the world
then my buds break open.

– C.G. Jung, *The Red Book*

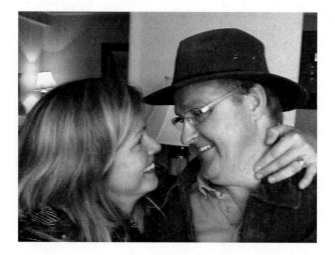

To Rob

Rob never declared that he was 'fighting' cancer.
Yet he lived every day in the hope that there would be
a tomorrow, until there simply wasn't.
When that time came, then he turned his face
to his end of life with a quiet courage that did not resist,
nor withdraw from us in despair or deny the inevitable.
He lived every day of his terminal illness with good humour
and love for his family. His dying was a full and rich living.
In his year of living with cancer, our witnessing this
was his tremendous gift to me and to all of our children.
I hope it becomes his gift to you.

— Jen

Contents

Foreword *by Judy Maddren*   xi
Introduction   xiii

Prologue   3
1 An Unlikely Pair   4

PART I   *Putting It Together*

2 The Shattering   15
3 The Team   22
4 The Updates   31
5 The Heartline   35

PART II   *Autumn 2009*

6 A Path Opens   49
7 What Will Death Look Like?   67
8 How Do We Do This?   80
9 We Make It to Christmas!   97

PART III   *Winter 2010*

10 From Sprint to Marathon   107
11 Rob Days   113

PART IV *Spring 2010*

12 Come Dance with Me   141
13 Tipping Point?   153

PART V *Summer 2010*

14 A Week at the Cottage   163
15 The Descent Begins   171
16 Feeling What He Needs   182
17 The Family Circle   197
18 Stay with Every Feeling   213
19 The Last Hurdle   223
20 Ten Days in September   230

Epilogue: How Do I Do This Alone?   251
The System and Us   273
The Authors' Own Stories   279
Acknowledgments   287
So What Is It Like Now?   293

Foreword

by Judy Maddren

Just Stay ... is a book with a predictable end, but the story that takes you there is probably nothing you could imagine. I could not put it down once I started reading.

Libraries and bookstores are full of 'how to' publications about health and life and dying. *Just Stay* ... is not a 'how to,' but a 'what if?' As with so many situations in our lives, if we only look at them another way, in a different light, we find a path through and discover unexpected gifts, as Rob and Jen Fazakerley did.

They immediately accepted the reality and finality of his diagnosis — metastatic cancer of the pancreas — in August 2009. But Rob and his caregivers, who included Jen, were able to shine another light, opening up possibilities for all of them as family, friends, and his health care team provided loving, hopeful care at home through his fourteen months with cancer.

Rob's experience offers us a perspective of hope — not the unrealistic dream of escape from disease and the continuing difficulties it presents, but hope in each day. Supporting him throughout were Jen, herself a community-care manager; Helen Butlin-Battler, a spiritual care specialist; and Grace Bradish, a nurse practitioner specializing in palliative care. They worked together with Rob, a physiotherapist, to ensure that it was his living that held meaning, not the cancer attacking his body.

IN MY YEARS as a national news broadcaster on CBC Radio and now as a personal biographer, I have learned that every life is remarkable. We have all needed to find courage, patience, and determination to get through tough times in our lives. We also know that the love and care of people who themselves offer patience and determination can make a real difference. *Just Stay...* is an enlightening and enlightened exploration of just such a partnership.

The story is also a reminder of the power of community. The book does not focus on Canada's system of health care, which provided and paid for the 'nuts and bolts' of Rob's physical care, although he and Jen were grateful for that. They both gave up their jobs when Rob became ill, but their employers and colleagues remained connected and supportive. Family, friends, and neighbours helped in many ways — most notably, in a community fund-raiser, 'Rob Fazakerley Day.' Regular, e-mail Rob Updates eventually reached thousands of readers, who sent notes, gifts, thoughts, and love. This wave of support buoyed Rob's spirits many times.

The e-mails, letters, and phone calls that flew back and forth between Jen, Helen, and Grace, as well as the Rob Updates, appear here in a kind of journal. They provide an intimate and absorbing view of Rob's illness, how it affected him and Jen and their family, and how the journey nourished each of them. The immediacy and the promising perspective of this narrative suggest the hope of 'what if?' and not the implacability of 'how to.' Ultimately, this is a reassuring story of a man's struggle with cancer and of the humanity and gifts of Rob and the people who loved and cared for him.

Introduction

Jen

WHEN YOU SET OUT to write a book, you presumably make a decision about what kind of volume you are writing. Is it a love story? A murder mystery? A thriller? A self-help guide? When the idea for this book first came along, I assumed it would be about grief, since only a few weeks had passed since my husband died. Now that Grace, Helen, and I have completed the manuscript, I realize this is a story about love and love's capacity to pierce through death.

This book was over two years in the making. It started without my knowing that it would ever become a book. It began in August 2009, when my husband, Rob, learned he had terminal pancreatic cancer. I am not alone in the awareness that cancer turns a family's world upside down. This is what happened to us.

I tell this story as Rob's wife and partner, and I feel confident that I can tell that part of the story very well. I know very well what it is like to look after a beloved spouse with a terminal illness, and I feel a personal connection to others who have walked that same path. I know what it is like to be a widow at age thirty-six. I cannot begin to understand what it is like to lose a father, a son, or a brother. Rob was all of those things to his family. In writing this story, I have focused almost exclusively on the interactions that took place between Rob and me. I felt that I had 'permission' to divulge those stories to the public, as they were my own. There was of course so much more that happened in that year than is contained in the pages of this book. Wonderful, laughter-filled, tender, heartbreaking moments between Rob and his children, Ben and Jessica, his parents, Brian and Mildred, and his brothers, Andrew, Malcolm, and Howard, not to mention my parents, John and Maureen Vickers, and my brother, John.

I cannot begin to imagine what it has been like for any of them to have travelled on this journey and would not presume to comment on their thoughts and feelings about their own experience. I know they all miss him terribly, and I have no doubt that the experience of knowing, and then losing, Rob has had a tremendous and lasting impact on their lives.

When Rob was diagnosed with cancer, I made a decision to leave my job and become Rob's primary caregiver for whatever short period we had left together. Within a very brief time, a team of health care providers gathered around us to help us in our journey.

It was in these early days that I came to meet two very important women, Helen Butlin-Battler and Grace Bradish. Helen is the spiritual care specialist at the cancer program where Rob received his treatment, and Grace is a nurse practitioner who provides care in people's homes. Over the course of Rob's illness, I was lucky enough to have these two wise women guide and support me through this treacherous territory.

Although Rob and I saw them both in person during counselling sessions with Helen and home visits by Grace, e-mail served as our primary method of communication. As Rob's illness progressed, I came to rely more and more on e-mail from each of them, both to sustain me spiritually and to maintain Rob clinically. It wasn't until after Rob died that I realized that they both had decided to keep all of the e-mails that we exchanged. They returned them to me and thus planted the seed of this book.

I have reflected a great deal on the wonderful gifts that came our way in the last year of Rob's life, and the most precious was perhaps the gift of a terminal diagnosis. Rob and I knew, and accepted, from the moment we learned it, that he would die from his disease. Knowing its terminal nature, and never allowing ourselves to play the 'one-in-a-million' game of hoping against hope for survival, forced us to clarify our priorities instantly.

If we had dared to feel even a slim hope for cure, it would have been so easy for us to wait for the 'go-ahead' to live each day as if it was our last day together. We did not do that. We always lived as if it was the last day. When I faced knowing I had only a very short time with Rob remaining, it made it very easy for me to suspend my career and focus my time and energy on him. It allowed us to make treatment decisions considering not slim survival statistics, but quality of life. It made it easy for Rob to focus on living and on enjoying his time to the fullest.

The world of cancer is full of encouraging messages of battle — "Cancer can be beaten," "Walk for the Cure," and "the fight against cancer." I certainly commend the tremendous strides that have taken place in cancer care and hope, for the sake of my own children, that this will be a disease of the past by the time they reach old age. Yet I wonder if this message of struggling against this disease has put a focus too strongly on curing and not strongly enough on living. A dying body has so few resources. I think Rob concentrated on simply living and did that brilliantly. He would often say, "Well, it is what it is," about any situation that we couldn't change while also doing everything possible to make the best of it.

Grace, Helen, and I tell this story in our three voices — a trio of women who experienced something life-affirming in Rob's illness and death. When we met, we were all health care professionals, and a wonderful man who faced cancer wove our lives together. We are now three women whose journey together has indelibly altered each of our lives.

This is a living story about the irrepressible forces of life, hope, and love that emerge so strongly even in death. Throughout Rob's illness, this journey seemed to draw in more and more people, changing their lives as they encountered Rob and the spirit in which he experienced not only his illness but also his life. This story wanted telling, perhaps so that it could keep finding people who need some soul food for their own difficult times. Perhaps this is why it has found you.

This book has truly been a collaboration. Helen and Grace and I are three very different women with three different voices, backgrounds, and histories, whose life-altering experience of supporting Rob through his illness and death transformed us. For me, I am so grateful that their support continued after Rob's death and expanded into a friendship that is foundational to this book. Preparing this volume required the unique talents and perspectives that each author brings.

Helen

THE STORY HAS, quite literally, compelled Jen, Grace, and me to write it. It began to take on its own life in late 2010 and early 2011 during a very long, cold winter. Does the world need another story about cancer? This was one question that concerned Jen and me as we began writing. Yet the story kept writing itself despite our questioning. *Something* wanted to surface.

In one layer, it is the personal, lived experience of Jen and Rob through their fourteen remarkable months of Rob's metastatic pancreatic cancer, which is a fatal diagnosis and to which he eventually succumbed. Yet the shattering is actually the beginning — it came with the diagnosis. The journey is a very different thing altogether. Far from being a terribly sad story, it tells us that, no matter how great the shattering, life can show up through the broken shards. How this happened lies in the moving account in the pages that follow.

Rob, Jen, Grace, and I were all health care professionals facing an intractable reality in Rob's diagnosis. Medical science and physical treatments of his cancer could not respond to it. The question his situation posed was clear: *How do I live when I know I am dying?* It is the razor-edge challenge for anyone living with a fatal diagnosis and confronts everyone involved in that journey. This was the question that animated Jen and Rob; Grace and I and the other professionals who threw themselves in with such total devotion experienced profound changes during our remarkable adventure with them.

My work in the cancer program has a depth and richness without parallel in my earlier years of hospital chaplaincy. I have been witness and guide to some of the most profound spiritual wrestling and transformation of people's lives within my small office and in hospital beds. Some days I have gone home feeling awe for the way life has a way of showing up for us. Some days I have left wondering what it all means and why such suffering happens.

But either way, every day, what I've experienced that day has challenged and enriched me. This has compelled me to keep diving into life and living myself. Every day. Little did Jen and Rob know, coming to me with their question, that they were giving me one of the most profound and unique journeys I have undertaken.

In my years in health care, I have encountered people's terror at suffering and death. I've witnessed and experienced how fear can be a cancer of the heart and mind that robs people of feeling alive and seen how its relentless grip prevents them from truly living in today. My work in the cancer program has evolved into developing *Soul Medicine,* which focuses on a 'targeted therapy for fear,' and fear has become my study.

Yet fear was not Jen and Rob's primary challenge. They did not come to see me because they were afraid, and that is what made this journey quite unusual. They came because they wanted to know, *How do we live this?* And thus the deep dive together began.

It is often the story of another person that nourishes us more deeply than the 'how-to's. Story reveals possibilities, and when we realize that there are, many possibilities in life, even in the face of death, then we take heart and summon the courage to continue with our own quest.

My hunch is that this is why this story is reaching out beyond Rob and Jen's immediate circle. This is not a religious or a scientific story, it is not about heroes and heroines battling cancer to the death. It is a story that we simply offer to you to let you see and feel that facing death, as painful as it is, is not the worst possible human experience. Many spiritual teachers have suggested this possibility, and I have witnessed its truth over and over again. Death is not the problem. Running from its reality is. This is the story of a courageous young couple who chose not to run.

This book started writing itself the day I offered Jen e-mail contact almost two months after we met. I'd never done this with anyone. It seemed the only way to keep in meaningful contact, as they lived outside London, and chemotherapy dominated their trips into town.

Had Jen not taken me up on this suggestion, we would not have captured this touching and transformative weaving of life and death in real time through our writing. Who knew we were writing to each other so that this could someday become nourishment for others' journeys? Who knew that Grace would also, simply on an instinct, keep all of her e-mails with Jen? Yet she did. This book was already taking shape unbeknownst to any of us. Rob and Jen's experience has changed Grace and me as much as anything that we offered and shared affected them. We followed our intuition as much as our skills in our roles as professionals and thus launched the process that we are now sharing with you.

For Jen and Rob, death was not a 'problem' to hurl their efforts against. They chose to not live their last months together in this physical life 'fighting cancer.' They certainly did everything medically possible to stave off its advance, but their inner attitude was not one of war or hope against hope. Instead they chose to let the awareness of its fatality guide them into living with every ounce of strength they had. They allowed death to thrust them into life and living. We have a health care system — one of the best and most technologically advanced in the world — that supports saving lives every day. Yet it has little to offer when life can no longer be 'saved' because it perceives death as 'the enemy.'

We seem as a society to have accepted a belief that we can and should stave off death at all costs and attempt to achieve painlessness as a way of life. We have forgotten that we must all face the great descent, and some of us sooner and more painfully than others. How do we prepare ourselves for this reality? How do we prepare our children? Jen and Rob faced these questions and tackled them head on.

Before I met them I had often seen how living with a confirmed fatal cancer can be treacherous and even sometimes spiritually annihilating, driving some people to despair, as they feel that their god or life has abandoned them. These deaths have been for me some of the most painful to witness.

Jen and Rob, in contrast, embraced the demands of keeping 'one eye on death and one eye on life' at all times to discover what might come of it. Both Grace and I marvelled at their ability to sustain this tension of opposites without collapsing on one side into despair or on the other into ungrounded hope. Through their living of this tension they allowed the powerful forces of life to break through. The opposites of life and death collapsed, taking them to a whole new place they had never experienced before. It did not erase the pain of it all, but it carried them in and through it all to a place where life, hope, and love could find them again and again and again.

And this is the very heart of this story. In a more encompassing way, beyond the personal details, it embodies an irrefutable truth that death never has to have the last word. Green shoots grow through the cracks in the concrete. Spring follows winter. This story reveals through lived experience that somehow, in some way, life can weave a 'new' through every apparent ending.

This was Jen, Rob, and their family's experience, and, judging by the circles upon circles of people who became involved and whom they somehow touched or changed, it has been this for many people along the way. As shattering as each ending may be, there are forever those invisible forces of life, hope, and love that somehow manage to create rebirth. No matter how deep the anguish or how much the heart is feeling pain, life's healing and potent renewing forces can work their magic.

After Rob's death, Grace, Jen and I came together in miraculous feats of scheduling that simply opened up in our very busy lives to remember and share our unique perspectives on the journey and began bringing them forth into narrative. Weekend after weekend, a deep current of energy pulled us together to bring this story into form and offer it to whomever we were writing if for — and we certainly knew not whom. Who would read this? We had no idea. We knew only that we were writing to share this with a future trail of people whom this story would find, one by one, in moments where they might most need this life-affirming experience.

And this is another layer of the story. It shows how the interior, intuitive path emerges like a silent river that carries us if we step in without resistance. This book conveys the organic essence of Rob and Jen's journey into the very heart of life. It is an offering to all those people facing soul pain beyond their comprehension as bread for the journey, one fellow pilgrim to another.

It takes tremendous courage to turn one's head towards pain, towards the reality of death when it comes knocking at one's door. Jen and Rob did this, and they discovered that not only were they living but also in many moments they were dancing. They were living the dance of their lives, astounding many people around them at how this was possible. What was their secret? They faced death and let it teach them how to live.

I am deeply grateful for the privilege of Jen, Rob, and Grace's weaving me into this journey. It is our great honour to share this journey with you.

Just Stay ...

Just Stay ...

Prologue

Jen

ON MY THIRTIETH BIRTHDAY I stand in my small hospital office. It is 8 October 2004. Rob hands me a long, rectangular box. "I've been a bad lad," he says with his best Liverpool Scouse accent. I open my gift. It is a white gold necklace with three pierced globes hanging from it. I put it on, and we hug and kiss (quite passionately for the workplace!), and then he dashes off to see his next patient for physiotherapy. I walk out of the office into the wide hallway, I had to tell someone. We are a couple! We are OUT as a couple.

SIX YEARS LATER in our bedroom in our beautiful house. Rob's parents, his children, his twin brother, he, and I are all in the bedroom. His breathing has stopped. His heart is still. It's one-thirty-five in the morning on 25 September 2010. I take his left hand in mine and straighten his fingers, still warm and pink, slip his wedding band off his hand, and string it onto the necklace that I received from him only six years earlier.

THIS BOOK is the story of the journey in between and beyond.

CHAPTER 1

An Unlikely Pair

∞

Jen

Rob and I had a wonderful marriage. We often used to talk about our incredible experience as 'us,' long before Rob was ill. We had both had another spouse — Rob for almost twenty years, I for just five. I think it was what we had gone through in relationships that had not worked that allowed us to approach our life together differently.

On the surface, we were a very unlikely pair. I have often told the story of my first meeting Rob, in 1999, one month after my first wedding. We met at a Human Dynamics seminar for which the hospital we were both working for had paid. Hospitals across Ontario were restructuring and amalgamating, and our administration had invested in team-building workshops to help smooth these transitions.

Human Dynamics is essentially a personality workshop where individuals answer a series of questions and respond to scenarios with the goal of determining their personality type. Ours lasted two days and took place in a conference centre. By midway through the first day many participants had begun to sort themselves into personality groups. Out of one hundred and fifty or so participants, I found myself in a group with only one other person. It was Rob. I had never met him before, although he was a fixture of St. Joseph's Parkwood Hospital in London, Ontario, as a physiotherapist who had been there for over twelve years.

My initial impressions of him focused on the physical. He was short, skinny, looked to be pushing forty, wore very unattractive shoes, and had a very outdated moustache. He also had a very engaging way about him, which was helped along considerably by his charming Liverpudlian accent. I was twenty-five, just shy of six feet tall, and blonde, and I had just married.

We spent the next two days together, just the two of us, in our apparently rare personality group. It was fascinating. The facilitator of the workshop walked the crowd through various problem-solving exercises to demonstrate how people who share a personality type also share their views on the world, their approach to challenges, their problem-solving strategies, and much more.

The two days filled up with rich conversation about everything under the sun. Rob was intriguing. He had moved to Canada from England in 1987 when he was just twenty-four. Parkwood Hospital had recruited him at a time when Canada was short of physiotherapists. He had grown up in Liverpool in a family with parents Brian and Muriel and brothers Andrew, Howard, and Malcolm, who was his own identical twin. He spoke fondly of his childhood — going to an all-boys school, sharing a small bedroom with two of his brothers, playing soccer and rugby, swimming competitively, and loving all things to do with sports.

Rob talked about Malcolm in particular. They shared their world, and I noticed he talked about growing up using 'our' instead of 'my' to describe things, such as 'our brother' and 'our mother,' as if he and his twin were one. They shared a bedroom until Malcolm went away to university, and they got up to all sorts of tricks. Clearly Rob loved playing jokes on people. He and Malcolm would switch places on their teachers and even on their family — and usually fooled everybody. Even buddies and girlfriends found themselves on the receiving end.

On a more serious note, Rob recalled an event when they were in their teens. He was downstairs talking with his mother and suddenly asked her, "What's wrong with Malcolm?" His brother was nowhere in sight. Before his Mum could respond, Rob ran upstairs to find Malcolm having a seizure. He told me that he had just known something was wrong. I asked him if he had some sort of mental connection with his identical twin, and he replied, "Of course," as if it was the air he breathed.

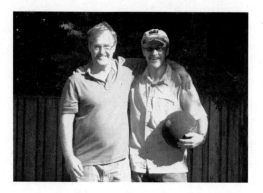

He reminisced about the adventure of coming to Canada from England and the challenge of leaving his family behind. He remembered the struggles and adventures of being a young father in a new country. He talked about how much he loved being a physiotherapist. He talked about his young children, Ben and Jessica, who took dance lessons and went to public school, and about their house in a small country village.

During our two days together, I told Rob about my recent wedding, my new house in the country, my university days, my parents, and my brother. We talked non-stop for two days. There was no hint of physical or sexual attraction between us, simply connecting (although years later Rob talked about how lucky he felt to be spending two days with a tall, blonde, twenty-five year old!).

I left feeling that this Human Dynamics stuff must be the most incredible personality tool ever, because I had clicked so strongly with this other person in my group. Of course, I now know that the click I experienced was not the magic of the personality seminar; it was the magic that Rob and I created together, it was just the wrong timing.

I also had a lingering, eerie feeling that I absolutely did not want to speak to Rob again if I saw him at the hospital.

It was as though in two short days I had opened up my soul and let him in. Well, in truth, I had. I had talked so openly with him during the workshop, with no filter on what I should or shouldn't say to this complete stranger. I told him what I really thought of my work and family, my hopes for the future, and my fears. Now I was going to run into this person at work. None of my colleagues knew these things about me, but he did. It made me feel uneasy, as if, when I saw him again, he would immediately get right into my head and read my mind. I'm sure that sounds crazy, but that feeling left me turning into side corridors or bathrooms whenever I saw him bounding down the hall. I avoided him like the plague for at least a year.

MY LIFE EVOLVED as lives do. I had my children — Jack and Haley — in quick succession just thirteen months apart. My professional life moved to the back burner as I took time off with maternity leaves and worked part time. I loved being a mother. I had a boy and a girl and was happy with that number of children.

Unfortunately, not all parts of my life were as fulfilling as motherhood. By the time I returned to work after my second maternity leave, I knew my marriage was coming to an end. Years later I can now reflect back and realize that this was a necessary step in the evolution of my life, but it was very hard — on me, on my husband, and on our youngsters. As Rob would probably say, "It was what it was."

My personal life was not something I openly shared at work. I had developed a few close friends there with whom I would talk openly about children, but nothing more. The demise of my marriage was private. I felt ashamed of it. I had been a wife for only four years and felt that I had failed. It was hard to admit to, and impossible to talk about.

At work, hospital restructuring continued, and everyone switched offices to accommodate new programs. The team I was part of — mostly my close friends — now shared a small office together, after having separate spaces previously. We all adapted.

My marriage continued to crumble, and I began to plan quietly and privately the logistics of separation. I went to work each day, and, without the benefit of walls between us, would put on a brave face and talk to my friends about the antics of my kids, by then one and a half and two and a half. It was then that a second team moved in with us — the Stroke Pilot Program — four more people cramming into the little office. One of them was Rob.

My heart sank. Immediately, I remembered the diving into corridors to avoid this person. This was going to be so uncomfortable. Rob was of course so cheery, so easy-going. I noticed he had aged considerably and seemed more serious. I convinced myself that perhaps things wouldn't be so bad. After all, we were both part of "outreach" teams that were in the community most of the time.

Yet within a couple of weeks Rob and I find ourselves one morning in the office à deux. I'm working on the computer, and he's writing chart notes at the desk behind me. There's an awkward silence.

"So, how are you, Rob? How are things with your kids? How is your wife?" I ask. I feel the need to ask so as not to appear rude.

"Oh, they're fine. Kids are fine. Jessica is still dancing. They're getting ready for her year-end show at the studio. Ben is figuring out what he's going to do in the autumn. He's supposed to start college in September. He's working at Zellers.

"Umm." He hesitates. "I'm not really sure how things are with my wife — she's in England. Things are not so good, I guess. How are things with you? How is your family?" he asks.

I stop typing and turn around. It is an absolute rule at Parkwood that people do not have, let alone discuss, marital problems. For four years I have not exchanged any more than formal pleasantries with this person sitting in front of me, and now he is divulging this? How do I respond to this level of honesty?

"Well, the kids are fine. Haley's walking now. Jack is in the terrible twos. My marriage has fallen apart. I'm trying to sort out how to separate." I respond with truth.

This is a crack in the wall. I have said things out loud. My emotions come welling to the surface, right there in our little office, and I quickly stuff them back down.

I can't remember the rest of what we said, but I know that we sat and talked about our crumbling and crumbled marriages for the next half-hour until Rob's next patient arrived. The conversation ended with his saying we should talk more over coffee, to which I readily agreed.

It felt a huge relief to be able to talk to someone about this darkness I was living in. Rob would later tell me that was also the first time he had said anything to anyone about his own marital problems and told me he felt a weight lifting off his chest. He told me it amazed him that I would listen to him talk about his problems. Of course the feeling was mutual.

We started meeting regularly for coffee in the cafeteria at Parkwood. Within a few weeks I had separated from Dave, and not long afterwards Rob's separation became final. We were each other's support group through this time. There was no attraction, no romance, nothing like that. A mutual respect was emerging, and we did a great deal of listening to each other and of understanding the pain we were each experiencing. We felt concern for each other's well-being and kept reassuring each other that things would be OK.

At some point over the next few months, chemistry developed between us. It was subtle at first, and I found myself doubting its presence, but it was there. One day we were talking over lunch hour at a local coffee shop. I found myself becoming quite upset talking about how difficult things were as a single mother of two young children. I was questioning whether I had made the right choice to leave my marriage and imagining the horrible impact that the divorce would surely have on my children, not to mention the financial and social implications.

I must have been quite a sight as we drove back to the hospital after lunch, tear stained and makeup running. As we were pulling into the parking lot, Rob reached across the gear shifter and took hold of my hand. I remember an electric jolt running up my arm the moment he took my hand. He stopped the car a few feet shy of the parking gate and turned to me.

"You'll be OK, Jen. You made the right decision. You're a good Mum, and your kids will be fine."

He looked deep into my eyes for just a few seconds, and my surroundings seemed to disappear. He had never held my hand, and I clearly remember thinking that he was a wonderful man, and I loved him. For a couple of months we had been talking almost daily about our lives, and I had come to look forward to our conversations, but before this second I hadn't had any romantic notions about this short, older Englishman with a moustache. How my life would change!

I have to say that after that moment our feelings for one another were rather like a freight train. Try as I might to put the brakes on and rationalize the hundreds of reasons why this wasn't a good idea (he's older than I, he's shorter, he has teenagers and I have toddlers, neither of us had formally divorced, and so on) nothing could stop us. We fell head over heels for one another.

Our friends and colleagues commented on how happy and young and full of life we both seemed. It was a wonderful time. Life had a lot of promise, and everything seemed so easy. It shouldn't have been easy. Rob and I were each going through the legalities of splitting up assets, finalizing custody arrangements, and working out agreements with our former spouses and therefore dealing with lawyers almost daily. We started to introduce our children to one another and navigate the complexities of dating while being parents of young and not-so-young children.

Rob's daughter, Jessica, was thirteen, and his son, Ben, was eighteen. The idea of their Dad's dating some strange woman certainly did not enthrall them. I tried my best. I took Jessica shopping and started attending her dance events. I took Ben to his college orientation and bought him beer. It was tough, however.

Haley and Jack adjusted more easily, as they were just two and three. I couldn't believe how wonderful Rob was with them. He would lie on the floor for hours playing blocks or Thomas trains or Tea Party. He knew how to use strollers and car seats and had numerous tricks for diffusing temper tantrums and bedtime arguments. He was a veteran Dad. The kids loved him.

After we had been together for a year, Rob and I took his children on a trip to England for me to meet his family. It was important to us that I meet his family, so off we went. Rob came alive in Liverpool. He was so excited to show me his roots. We met up with several of his boyhood friends. He introduced me to each of them with a huge grin, "This is my girlfriend, Jen."

I've never had so many people eye me up and down as in those three weeks in England! An unlikely pair we may have been, but I have since heard that everyone could see how much we were in love.

IT WAS SHORTLY AFTER we returned from England that Rob and I started talking about marrying. It was still a distant goal, but it had entered our conversations. Rob would always say, "When we get married," not "If." We both felt we had to signal to our children that there was serious, unwavering commitment between us, and marriage seemed a logical way to do it.

At Christmas 2005, Rob gave me a gold Celtic ring. "I wish I could ask you to wear this on your left hand, but perhaps, for now, put it on your right." I wore the ring on my right hand until March, when we started looking for houses. After a few weeks of looking, we found our home — a beautiful, yellow-brick, mid-Victorian five-bedroom house in atrocious condition. Perfect! A project! The day we put the offer in, Rob asked me to move my ring over, and it became my engagement ring.

Bringing our families together in our new home was a monumental task. Ben and Jessica resisted at first, but we soldiered on. We gave each of them a hefty decorating budget for their own spaces and open access for their friends at any time. Our house soon became a busy place, with at least one friend at the dinner table most nights. Slowly we developed a routine and adapted to one another.

Rob and I were so incredibly happy. We loved being with each other. We were a couple of homebodies, spending most of our free time in our home, fixing it, painting and decorating it, planting beautiful English gardens, and talking long into the night. Rob was so handy around the house; he could fix just about anything and had a huge capacity to do so. We loved working on the house, we made a great team, doing everything together. We were very compatible, whether we were painting a living-room, building a patio, parenting a four-year-old, or teaching a teenager to drive.

At work too we loved to be together. I found watching Rob doing his physiotherapy with patients absolutely riveting. I came to realize that his professional reputation had spread far and wide. Other therapists would often call him for his opinion about clinically challenging patients. He might say, "Oh, I'll just pop up and see them on my lunch hour."

He'd meet these patients, often frail and elderly, and spend a few minutes just talking with them. He would then take their hand, perhaps examine a foot, and next, with a few, well-placed fingertips on back and shoulders, would manage to ease people into standing, even walking, after only a few minutes and what appeared to be a very minimal assessment. He was famous for this. New and seasoned therapists would stand watching this interaction, slack-jawed, and comment, "I've been working with that lady for *four months,* and she's never done that!" It was magical to watch.

Rob and I never really fought, although we had many, many discussions about everything. We made a deal with one another at the very beginning of our relationship that we would tell each other everything, particularly what the kids said to each of us about the other. It wasn't always easy to hear, but we stuck with this deal and extended it to all parts of our relationship. I think back now and believe it was probably our communication challenges in our first marriages that spurred us to change everything in our second.

WE MARRIED ON 22 October 2006, after being together for about two years. We held the ceremony in our dining-room in front of forty relatives and friends. Rob's family stayed with us — ten people in total. Rob was in his element. He was able to show his family his new house, his new town, his new little step-kids, his new big family, and his bride. We had a fun day, with lots of laughter, despite the dreary late-October weather.

We packed a lot into the next three years. We continued our house projects, and we took family camping holidays, trips to Florida (including, of course, Disney World), a wonderful holiday in the Caribbean, and another back in England for Rob's parents' fiftieth wedding anniversary, and we had lots of short weekend excursions away with and without the kids.

We both made some career changes. I left the security of Parkwood Hospital and went to the South West Community Care Access Centre (SWCCAC) as a project manager and then a regional manager. Rob moved from stroke to spinal-cord rehabilitation, and then finally to the Community Stroke Rehabilitation team, an outreach program that had emerged from the pilot project in which he had been working when we found ourselves sharing the same office.

Rob was a tremendous support to me. He was proud of my successes at work. We shared the household tasks equally. He did the laundry, I prepared the meals, he took on the vacuuming, and I did the dusting. We both picked up kids and dropped them off at baby sitters, dance classes, and school programs.

We would often say to each other, in the busy days of family life, things like, "We're so lucky, we love each other so much." "What a great marriage." "What would we ever do without one another?" We were very close, respected each other tremendously, and loved each other very deeply.

Part One

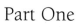

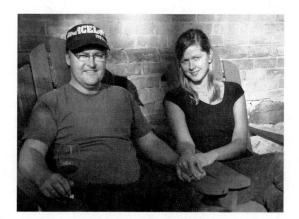

Putting It Together

CHAPTER 2

The Shattering

∞

Monday 10 August 2009
Diagnosis

Jen

BLOOD WORK AT Tillsonburg District Memorial Hospital in early August reveals that Rob's liver enzymes are very high and climbing.

Learning this terrifies me. This can't be good. Some doctor along the way has learned of our professions in health care. "Perhaps Rob has acquired hepatitis?" he wonders aloud. It doesn't add up, however. It is the wrong set of symptoms, but it is a better alternative than where my mind is taking me.

Doctors order more tests, including a CT scan in London on 7 August. That day arrives, and I go to work. I'm a wreck. I know something is terribly wrong, I can feel it in my bones. I leave a meeting crying and go straight home to be with Rob. He is home from the scan, and he looks exhausted, pale, and grey.

By the following Monday (the 10th) we are both in the emergency room at Tillsonburg Hospital. I drive us that morning after a sleepless night of Rob being in pain. Rob doubles over in the car in agony. The trip seems endless, although it takes less than twenty minutes.

They see Rob immediately. The results from the previous Friday's scan are in. The emergency room physician comes to us. Rob is on a gurney, covered in a white sheet, looking so small.

"Do you have any cancer in your family?" the doctor asks, holding the chart against his chest.

Rob looks at me, and he can't find words.

Oh, no, I think, horrified. But my mind for details steps in and takes over.

"Yes, his paternal grandfather died of pancreatic cancer in his fifties, as well as other types of cancer in all his other grandparents." I rattle off the information while another part of me, inside, is crumpling. "I believe his Mum had some early cancer detected after a stomach surgery, as well, which was removed surgically."

There is a long pause.

The doctor is reading and re-reading the chart.

"The CT scan results are back. It looks like a tumour. Cancer, in the pancreas," he pauses, "and it looks like it's spread to the liver."

Rob reaches up to hold my hand. Tears spring from his eyes. My head is buzzing, my throat aching, I can't breathe properly. My husband, my dear, beloved Rob, who is only forty-six, has metastatic pancreatic cancer. My mind scans rapidly. What do I know about this? It doesn't take long to find the data in my memory.

It is a death sentence.

I know it kills people very fast. I know it is supposed to be a horrible, painful cancer. All this I recall in less than a second or two.

And I know in the glaring light of the emergency room that I will lose him.

"Oh, Rob! I love you. Oh, no!" I sob. I am in utter disbelief. I look down, awkwardly trying to hold him while he is lying on the gurney.

The physician reminds us of his presence: "Do you have any children?"

"We have four." Rob replies quietly.

"Well, we have to act fast," insists the doctor. "This is an aggressive type of cancer. We will get a referral into the cancer clinic in London to have you seen as soon as possible. For now, we will have you seen by one of our internists here after we've admitted you. And maybe we'll see about getting you some privacy in the meantime."

Another pause, then he adds, "I'm so sorry, Rob."

He leaves.

Rob needs to use the bathroom. I take the minute while he is there to call one of my dearest friends, who is also a doctor — Julia. I'm sobbing almost uncontrollably from a bathroom stall.

"Julia, I'm in Tillsonburg Hospital. Rob's just been told he has pancreatic cancer that has spread to his liver."

"Oh, no, Jen!!! Oh, noooo!!" Her wail down the phone is piercing.

She sobs, loudly. "Jen, I'm so sorry." She is not the calm physician in this moment. She is my dear friend, our dear friend, as gutted as we are.

Her cry gives me all the information that nobody has yet offered us, but that I already suspect. This is the death sentence I think it is.

"Julia, how long?"

"Oh, Jen. Metastatic pancreatic cancer? Three to six months at best." Her ability to be clear and truthful, knowing that nothing less will do any good, comes to the fore.

Rob appears from the bathroom and heads to the gurney.

"OK, Julia. I have to go. Rob's back at his bed. Bye."

My beloved, my soulmate. I would have him for what? Three more months?

My whole world's collapsing.

Tuesday 11 August 2009
Tillsonburg Hospital

Jen

"How BIG IS IT?" Rob wants to know. He's lying in his bed on the medical unit at Tillsonburg Hospital. This is his second day there, and he's getting Demerol injections for his acute pain. The medical staff is trying hard to wrestle the pain under control.

"The tumour, you mean?" I ask.

"Yes."

"Well, it's two-point-nine centimeters by three-point-two centimeters" — my mind for details has them all trapped and lined up.

Rob and I had both long believed his symptoms were the result of 'something like an ulcer' from the diffuse symptoms he had, which is a very common misdiagnosis with pancreatic cancer. Current belief is that this cancer starts and spreads quickly — it's not a slow-growing form — but I've been mentally searching for clues of when this started and wondering how long Rob has been living with this growing in his body. Hindsight is of course twenty/twenty. When I think back now to the year preceding Rob's cancer diagnosis I realize there were subtle changes in his health at least six months before that. He had always had "stomach problems."

At the very beginning of our relationship he had an emergency appendectomy secondary to acute abdominal pain. After the operation, the surgeons found out they had just removed a completely healthy appendix and had no explanation for the acute pain. They had inspected Rob, quite literally, from one end to the other, and they had uncovered nothing. They labelled him with gastro-esophageal-reflux disease (GERD), prescribed Panteloc to reduce the acid, and told him to eat more fibre. He did that, and for five years he appeared to be fine.

The old familiar 'stomach' problems, however, started to resurface around Christmas 2008. He had vague pain and, occasionally, nausea. I didn't pay much attention and, in fact, became a bit annoyed at his complaints, because I thought the discomfort the result of a lapse in his high-fibre diet.

The complaints came and went over the winter but were becoming more consistent in April. By June, he was having quite a lot of pain at night and started to elevate his head and chest before sleep. He arranged a doctor's appointment for vacation time in early July, so he wouldn't have to miss work. He was still doing jobs around the house, but he seemed to drag himself around and seemed noticeably tired.

In my gut I knew something was wrong by late May. I really worried and started doing research on the internet. I wondered about something in his pancreas, because of some specific complaints about his bowels and appetite. I tried to put the worry out of my head but found it consumed me.

Tenderness developed between us over the summer as I think we both came to realize that whatever this was it was probably serious. Rob later told me that he suspected pancreatic cancer in July after reading about the symptoms over my shoulder when I was looking at things on the internet. He hadn't said anything, knowing he had a doctor's appointment in a couple of weeks.

In the middle of July 2009 we took a vacation. We packed up and took Jack and Haley to the Pinery Provincial Park for a camping trip. Rob was clearly sick. I knew it. He knew it. He didn't want to cancel our holiday, although we talked about it. He went, I'm sure, for the kids, but it must have been so hard for him.

By late July and in the first few days of August, Rob had two trips to the emergency room at Tillsonburg Hospital and a family doctor's appointment, all in response to increasing pain.

There was a sombre, heavy feeling around our house. Each time he went into the emergency room the doctors ordered tests and blood work. It all came back ominous: "There was something on the ultrasound." "Your liver enzymes are elevated; maybe it's hepatitis, maybe it's gall-stones, maybe it's something a bit more sinister." "We'll order a CT scan in London."

In the medical unit, my mind is reeling. I know that keeping track of the details is now my job. Details can lead to fatal mistakes if they disappear between charts and providers.

"So, about this big?" Rob holds up his hand in an approximation of the size.

"Yes, like that," I respond, snapped back to the present.

"So, about the size of a golf ball?" Rob is heading somewhere with this, but I'm not sure where. "Well, that's not that bad," he states simply, purposefully.

WHAT? It's huge! I think to myself. Reading the CT report the day before — at my own insistence — had stunned me. This cancer must have been growing inside him for ages to reach this size. The doctor had let me read the document while he hovered over my shoulder.

Rob continues, pondering his imaginary golf ball. "Well, we'll just have to do something about that," he states, an upbeat canter in his voice.

"OK." I respond, wondering how exactly that is going to happen. Knowing it likely won't. For the thousandth time that day, tears well up in my eyes. "It's OK," Rob says.

He is so calm.

I am in pieces.

I don't know anything about the diagnosis or prognosis other than it is terminal. I don't know how we are going to tell the kids and how they will ever handle this. My career is suddenly hanging on a thread, stopped short and flailing in the wind. All I know is that I am leaving it and hoping maybe I'll have a job to return to. I have no spiritual connection to anything — no church, no minister to tell me everything will be OK or to comfort me with whatever ministers comfort people with.

We have just married, less than three years ago. We have so many plans — we do lots of planning, and we always have projects on the go. We've renovated our house, and there's more to do — a joy for both of us. Now, suddenly, all these plans are like a road falling off a cliff with landslide, and we're free falling. I don't know what the treatment will be, who our team is. There is no team. I feel absolutely at sea. I feel like I have to carry it all. I don't know if I can, but I have to for Rob's sake, I have to.

Wednesday 12 August 2009

Jen

WE'VE BEEN HOME a few nights. I have a dream.

I am in a large, open-air, hospital-type place, like how I imagine a hospital would be in a war or in a third-world country. Water surrounds it — in my dream representing the Mersey River — and in my dream this is Liverpool (where Rob grew up). There are rickety, narrow, steep stairs everywhere, all made of wood. There are archaic escalators with railings that sink into the floor at the top and bottom where they meet the floor.

It is cold and wet. Rob and I have come to this place to find a doctor. He is very sick and weak. I have my arm around him, and we are walking out towards a large, semi-circular balcony overlooking the river, with a low railing along the edge. We approach the doctor and begin speaking to him. He is standing at the balcony's edge.

Rob then tells me he is going to be sick. I rush to the edge with him, and he throws up over the side. I see a friend (an old colleague from Parkwood Hospital) and ask her to bring me a glass of water. She runs with this glass, but slips, and ends up falling into the water. Rob is anxious about her. She is obviously hurt but says she is fine.

As the commotion clears, we look around, and the doctor has gone. We see him far away in an upper balcony, accessible only by many flights of stairs. I look at Rob — he is so sick and weak, and I know I need to carry him. I pick him up like you would a small child. His eyes have closed, and I start walking to reach this doctor. As I look down at Rob in this dream, it amazes me that I can carry him. He is not heavy.

As I navigate up and rickety, wobbly stairs. I worry so much I will drop him, but I don't. I go up the escalator. My skirt catches in the railing going into the door. I still don't drop him. I climb up a very difficult, steep set of stairs almost to the top, only to reach a barricade that I can't hop over carrying Rob — and I will not put him down.

Finally, I reach the upper balcony. Several doctors are sitting chatting. The one we met earlier stands up and faces us. I say, "We left before you finished what you were saying," and he replies, "Oh, I was just going to say that there's nothing we can do for your husband."

The dream is true.

Friday 15 August 2009

Jen

ONE NIGHT, LATE, I can't sleep at all. It's five days since the diagnosis. I feel completely ripped open. Weeping as I drop to my knees in the living-room, I am begging for more time.

I feel hands settling on my shoulders and a calming presence saying: "It's OK, you've got time." And my tears stop.

I feel strangely peaceful for brief moments for the first time since the diagnosis.

CHAPTER 3

The Team

⌒⌒

Jen

WITHIN A FEW WEEKS of Rob's diagnosis, our team falls into place: the palliative care doctor, the oncologist, the nurse practitioner, and the spiritual care specialist.

The Palliative Care Doctor

Jen

DR. KAREN FRYER, the palliative care physician for our area of Oxford County, comes to our home to meet us on Tuesday 18 August. She is young, much younger than I had expected. She's very kind and warm, and her presence is a comfort. Rob is in bed today. He's very sick. I lead her upstairs to see him.

Rob looks extremely tired, truly worn. She introduces herself to him, and I notice that she is very gentle, kind, and soft-spoken. I have liked her from the first time I talked to her on the telephone, and we have already had several phone chats. Rob's pain has been out of control, and she has been working with us on it very skilfully.

She examines him. I sit on the bed beside him, and then she sits in a chair next to the bed on the other side of him.

I ask her the question that is sitting over us like a black crow, silent but present. "Can you tell us what to expect? What prognosis do you expect?"

"Metastatic pancreatic cancer is terminal, and you need to be thinking in terms of weeks to months. You should be getting your affairs in order, Rob," she responds, speaking gently.

Weeks? is my first thought. Never has it occurred to me that it might be only weeks.

But she goes on, "Having said that, I have no idea of the impact of chemotherapy, I am not the oncologist. I am the palliative care physician."

She would see us at home about every two weeks.

The Oncologist

Jen

WE MEET WITH THE ONCOLOGIST on Monday 31 August, at the busy London Regional Cancer Program.

We ask him the same question: "How long do you anticipate we have?"

He turns the question back to us: "What are you hoping for?"

Rob says, "We have four children, so I'd like to be able to make it to Christmas. I know its terminal, but I'd like to be able to see Christmas. Well, for that matter," he adds with a rueful grin, "I'd like to be able to see lots of Christmases, but ..." his humour surfacing, even now.

The specialist replies, "Well, I think that's reasonable. I think we can probably get you to Christmas." I can almost see him counting on his hands how far away that event is. Sixteen weeks — four *months*.

We feel some flicker of hope. It is the first flicker since the diagnosis. Maybe we'll have more time than we've thought.

I tell the doctor, "When we'd walked in, I was afraid you'd say, 'We can't offer you anything, this is pancreatic cancer.'" I am checking him out a little bit. For my own reassurance, I need to hear that this is what he is *not* saying. I'll take any crumb at this point.

"Oh, well, there's always hope," he responds, with an assurance that is comforting. He continues, "You just have to know what to hope for. You hope for tomorrow."

We're down to tomorrows. While comforting, it solidifies the reality of death coming and our awareness. It is a question of how we do this. I know it's not curable; this is going to end with Rob's dying. So what does "hope for tomorrow" actually mean when someday those tomorrows will end with Rob's death?

We had both worked professionally with many people who had suffered terrible brain injuries and strokes and catastrophic, life-altering health issues. We had both burrowed away on the subterranean level of people's lives on the elusive issue of hope. Hope for our various patients might mean living in a wheelchair, but not dying. Or having to let others bathe them and feed them, but still being able to see their children and grandchildren. Rob was famous for his ability to sustain hope for and with people when their situation seemed hopeless.

What does hope mean for us now?

The Nurse Practitioner

Grace

IT IS WEDNESDAY 2 September 2009, and I have just started on 4 August as a nurse practitioner at the Community Care Access Centre for the Southwest Region of Ontario in London, having left my position at the London Regional Cancer Program (LRCP).

I learn about a new patient, Rob, and his wife, Jen, whom I am to go and visit. They are a young couple who have just received a diagnosis of pancreatic cancer with metastasis to the liver. He's palliative from the get-go. He has had a pain crisis that the community palliative care physician resolved medically, and I have her report on her contact with them and his status. It's not good. And they're so young, with a young family. Another tough one.

My role is to educate them on chemotherapy expectations, coordinate his care with the LRCP, and direct them to the right people and places when issues arise.

The drive to their home is beautiful. They live in a lovely area in a small village, and the sun is shining today. It's refreshing, and I appreciate this benefit of my new job. I actually have a chance to see the fields and life happening outside the LRCP and my small office there.

I arrive at the lovely old house. It is warm and welcoming, and I use the front door, respecting the age-old tradition of not presuming oneself into people's lives through the back door.

Rob is sitting on their couch in the living-room. Jen is next to him. He looks relatively well; he has a good colour and is interactive and engaging. Jen is clearly the driver of his care and is asking really good and clear questions. I can tell she's done her reading on this. Rob, I notice, is very comfortable with letting her take that role. I can see the close relationship they have.

This is not always the case with patients. Sometimes people resist changes in roles, or old, unresolved rocks in the relationship rise up and smash them apart, making the whole thing so much more painful. Cancer does not always bring people closer together; it can tear families, relationships apart. I've seen it all.

Hearing Rob and Jen so open with me about their process so far, my gut tells me that this will likely be quite an incredible journey, however we do it. Their honesty, openness, and mutual respect are real strengths, which they will need. I am glad and relieved they have all this going for them.

We discuss chemotherapy, pain, and symptoms, their angst in anticipation of the chemotherapy, the side effects, what to expect in terms of benefit. I explain that the first cycle shows the patient's tolerance for it and the following two or three reveal if it's going to affect the cancer.

I examine Rob, hands on, to determine the baseline. As I do so, I am taking in how incredibly brave and courageous they are about the diagnosis and being so much in the present. It's pretty rare.

Thankfully, he can have chemotherapy — not always an option with metastatic pancreatic cancer if it has advanced too far. I can see how they want to make use of all the tools available.

They are also preparing to take Jessica, Rob's daughter, to university this week. We talk a fair bit about that, because I've just sent a daughter off to university — a personal connection I can meet them with.

I notice another personal link arising, one that I don't talk about —

it's much harder and more tender. My dear friend Carole flashes into my mind. Carole, or 'T,' as I affectionately called her, died of cancer two and a half years ago, and I still miss her a great deal. My good friend Betti's husband had died of cancer three weeks later. I did so much of their journey with both of those couples. I was their bridge with the health care system.

The similarities are hitting me hard in Jen and Rob's living-room. Their kids are all of similar ages. I know that this is a very, very painful process in every way. These couples who were my friends were also very close, strong, and aligned, and I look at Rob and Jen thinking, "This is another Carole and Steve or Matt and Betti," because they too never shied away from reality. I can feel the mix stirring of their sadness, loss, and grief, and my own grief. This too is part of the personal impact of our jobs in health care.

AFTER THE INITIAL VISIT, I contact Helen, the LRCP's spiritual care specialist, to seek support for myself as much as for Jen and Rob. We caregivers find that those personal and professional experiences of deaths that touch us deeply never disappear for us. We encounter them again and again when we meet similar situations. And cancer has taken so many of our friends and neighbours. It's prevalent. The personal is the professional, and the professional is personal.

I know this is going to be a big journey for all of us. My instincts say Rob and Jen need to meet Helen. My instincts also tell me, *I want the support in this one.* It's not going to be easy for anyone — I know all too well what lies ahead.

Jen

GRACE IMMEDIATELY impresses me. She has a calm competence that allows me to lower my guard. I feel that she won't let us down, that she will help us through. She looks to be somewhere around Rob's age and is very unassuming. From behind her glasses, her striking, sparkly eyes lock onto mine as we talk, and she has an open, expressive face. She looks like she could jump in and help in any emergency, and her practical and pragmatic air suggests she will just do whatever is necessary with absolute competence.

She speaks to us in a straightforward way, instinctively matching her descriptions of Rob's upcoming cancer treatment to our current level of knowledge and our intellects. What strikes me is how attentively she listens to Rob and me. She listens, and appears to believe us, as we describe our last three weeks and our observations of Rob's health.

Grace gives us more specifics about the drug Rob will be receiving in chemotherapy, but also takes time to ask about our children, Rob's family in England, and us. She mentions she lives on a farm and has horses that she loves, that her work takes her out into the country to places like ours. She tells us that she has two children about Ben and Jessica's age, which reassures me that she can appreciate the impact of this cancer on our lives. I feel a good connection with her.

Her parting line: "This is palliative care, but this is not end-of-life care. You have a lot of living left to do, and I'll try and help you feel well enough to do it." She planned to visit us every two weeks — so different from waiting hours in the clinic for a short time with the doctor. Thank goodness we live in a small community outside the city.

Rob comments after she leaves that he likes Grace. Having worked with many, many nurses over a long career in health care, he knows, without being judgmental or critical at all, whom he clicks with right away. As do I. Grace clicks. I feel relief after she leaves; she seems very knowledgeable about the cancer and the treatments, and she seems very human.

Grace is a perfect name for her. She's an oasis of comfort in this moment, and her visit to our home makes such a difference. Very quickly, she appears to have grasped who we are and what we are all about.

Our health team is coming together.

The Spiritual Care Specialist

Helen

"HELLO, HELEN, IT"S GRACE." The date is Wednesday 2 September 2009.

"Hi, Grace, how are you?" I reply. "Good to hear your voice. How is it out there in Community Care Access Centre land?"

I miss Grace at work. She was the nurse practitioner on my hiring committee four years ago. That interview marked my return to work, part time, as a hospital spiritual care specialist after my attempt to be a stay-at-home mother. I missed my work. I missed walking with people in the liminal places between life and death, where so much richness and life lie hidden.

My mandate when I started at the London Regional Cancer Program (LRCP) was to develop an outpatient model of spiritual care — it was no easy task finding the people who want or need spiritual support without being able to go and see them in their hospital beds.

For four years I have been building a referral-based spiritual care service for people living with cancer, referred from the front lines by various clinicians. Grace was one of the medical professionals who really understood what spiritual support could give people in the throes of cancer and that it does not mean religious rites only.

Many people are not part of any spiritual tradition yet have a strong desire to find some way of finding what trust means, what hope means, and how to live with their mortality fearlessly ... especially when cancer hits their lives. I have been learning much from countless people in their deep, soul-searching struggle of living with cancer and dying with it. Slowly, through listening to their experiences, I was discovering that cancer could be a powerful teacher and lead to profound spiritual resilience. It seemed often to ignite a potent awareness of the preciousness of life and a desire to live fully with whatever time remains.

Grace was very kind when I started and had given me a hand of friendship in a tough environment. She was one of three superb nurse practitioners in our program. I greatly missed her pragmatic, salty-humoured attitude, alongside her quiet expertise, when she left LRCP to work in community care.

I am very glad to be hearing her voice in the midst of this busy day. I settle back into my chair to focus fully on our conversation.

"It's going fine, Helen," she says, in answer to my question. "Really well. Crazy paperwork, as usual. I still don't have dictation capacity, if you can believe that? I have to do my notes by hand, and I'm way behind, you know. Anyway, we soldier on."

It's the same old story in health care — the juggling of all the administration that underlies our patient-care and front-line roles. Grace never wastes time dwelling on this; her focus on her patients is resolute.

"I just met a young couple, Helen, in the community, who I think need to see you. He's just been diagnosed with pancreatic cancer. He's young, only mid-forties, and she's even younger, in her mid-thirties. It's their second marriage; they have two young children who are from Jen's first marriage, eight and seven, and two older children of Rob's from his first marriage, late teens and early twenties.

"Rob is a physiotherapist at Parkwood Hospital, and Jen is a regional manager in Community Care Access Centre. It's devastating news for them, and they're just reeling. He's coming in for chemotherapy this week; do you think you could see them?"

I always trust the gut of people who refer patients to see me. Trying to discern spiritual needs is an art form that is very hard to teach. Grace is someone whose instincts I trust implicitly.

"Absolutely. When are they coming?"

"His chemotherapy is this Friday, September fourth, at noon." Grace, ever on top of the details, rattles off the information.

"Great, that's when I am working, and I'm open at noon." I note the serendipitous flow of this. My schedule is now often completely full. "That's great. I'll see them then and let you know how it goes."

"Thanks a lot, Helen. They're really going to need support. This is one of those really sad cases; life expectancy for pancreatic cancer is only a few months, if that. And I know, for myself, it is reminding me so much of my friend Carole, who died a couple of years ago, and soon after another couple who we were really good friends with, he died. I was really involved in both of their processes. I know I might need some support in this one, too. I'll send you a copy of their notes."

"I'm always here, Grace. Know that. We need each other in this work." A fact I've learned in great depth over four years of front-line cancer care. "Call anytime. We'll see what happens on Friday when I meet them, and I'll let you know."

"Great — thanks, Helen," Grace responds. I can feel the sense of shared support that linking with one another in these heart-wrenching cases gives us as professionals. We need that.

"You take care, Grace."

"You too, Helen."

I hang up, glad for the albeit-brief chance to reconnect with a good colleague, her competence always making the people around her feel they're on solid ground, including me.

I think again about how professional and personal intertwine in cancer care. This struck me when I began working at LRCP. More than anywhere else I'd worked, here friends, neighbours, and relatives might become our patients. Also, our cases frequently remind us of our own losses. Cancer is a shared experience in our society, gripping and affecting us all.

A sad and difficult journey lies ahead. I may need Grace too in this one.

CHAPTER 4

The Updates

❧

Sunday 30 August 2009

Jen

THE LAST TWO WEEKS we've had medical appointments daily. We're also trying to manage Rob's pain and symptoms — an enormous task.

The phone is ringing constantly — ten times an hour, it seems. Relatives in England and Canada, colleagues from Parkwood Hospital, friends — and everyone is saying, "Oh, my goodness, I just heard, how are things going?" Then they call back within a few days: "How are things going?" We are incessantly updating people between appointments and trying to process what has happened.

There are not enough hours in a day to deal with the appointments, Rob's symptoms, his needs, and the updating over and over and having to tell the story to fresh ears. It all seems brutal and exhausting. My children have gone to their father's place, thankfully, so I can focus totally on this and Rob.

Many callers also offer endless advice from their own experience with cancer in friends and colleagues. This is annoying, unsettling — and irrelevant. None of them has dealt with metastatic pancreatic cancer, and I feel like I'm doing a PhD reading up on it. I'm 'fast tracking' in the knowledge base, and it is expanding daily.

I have become Rob's protector from the outside world, and I am 'reading' him at any given moment to gauge his energy and capacity. We've only a short time together, and it's painful for him to keep explaining and reliving. I need to guard the little time he has left for living.

After two weeks of the incessant phone calls and requests for information, it's clear to me I have to come up with a communication plan. I tell Rob about the calls, but he is not able to absorb much information because he is so very sick. Friends and acquaintances often want to talk to Rob — if I let them, it's only for a couple of minutes.

Some folks have suggested many of the new electronic ways to communicate — blogging, care pages on the web. These just don't feel right for us. They are too public, and this is a very private experience. The public domain of the web feels like the wrong place to share all the details to update people.

ONE MORNING ROB is feeling unwell, and the phone has rung six times before ten a.m. I see my BlackBerry, my work device, on the kitchen counter. I fire off an e-mail to Monique, our dear friend and Rob's boss in the past year.

In the midst of all this, Monique has, unbeknownst to me, contacted my Mom to ask if there was anything she could do to facilitate better communication for us. Monique has a background in social work and is the new coordinator for the stroke program where Rob worked. My mother told me in an e-mail about Monique's question. Mom said to her, "Any amount of communication will be Jen and Rob's call. There's no script for this."

Here is Monique's way to help. I start writing to her about where we are at. I ask her to forward it to a close group of friends at Parkwood Hospital — Rob's colleagues — to keep them in the loop and reduce calls (about a quarter of them, as it turns out). I update her on Rob's status, and Monique becomes an invaluable updater on our process, saving us oodles (a nonscientific unit) of energy.

Wednesday 2 September 2009
First Rob Update

Rob was seen by an oncologist at London Regional Cancer Program on Monday, August 31. He will be starting palliative chemotherapy on Friday. He will have a chemotherapy drug called gemcitabine. Thank goodness for Canadian universal health coverage! This drug would cost us $1000 a week if we had to pay! It is not curative and has minimal impact on length of life, but is supposed to improve quality of life; namely decreasing pain, increasing energy, and decreasing nausea.

He will get chemotherapy intravenously once a week at London Regional Cancer Program for three weeks, then a week off, and then repeat these 'rounds' or 'cycles' as many times as he can. It will have side effects, but comparatively mild compared to other chemotherapies. We'll have to see how he reacts. Please pass on and also pass on our sincere thanks for the wonderful cards, food, and best wishes e-mails.

Thanks

Jen

Wednesday 2 September 2009

Jen

WITHIN HOURS of sending this note, I receive thirty e-mail responses. It is so much better: none of them asks for information — they already have that — and they offer support, food, meals, child care, and lawn care and send us good wishes, which are very heartening.

I take my BlackBerry into the living-room and start reading them to Rob, and, as I read, more are coming in. They are a deluge of love and care. They are so instantaneous, and what a different feeling from the phone calls, which seem so intrusive. They allow us control over how and when we respond.

The updates evolve as time goes on and become a lifeline between Rob and me and our outside world. The distribution list expands with each one.

We ask Monique (always the gateway) to add people as word of Rob's diagnosis creeps into wider circles of our lives. Still, friends and colleagues from Rob's past find out and call us, and we start from the beginning, with diagnosis, and so on — but now we can invite them to join the e-mail list. They always accept.

A pattern emerges: I send an update, often after our monthly appointment with the oncologist. Rob and I talk about what information to include, I write a draft, I review it with Rob (while sitting on the couch with my BlackBerry), and he edits it for content. I send it out to Monique, who then forwards it to the 'ethers.' Within five days our mailbox — that is, our Canada Post box in Norwich — fills with cards. My e-mail inbox overflows. It is overwhelming.

"People are so kind. I can't believe how many people are thinking of me. I'm just Rob," he says, shaking his head in disbelief. "Everybody is pulling for me. I guess I'd better keep going!" he jokes. Always his good humour. It's so humbling, so heartbreaking.

I think, *Well, of course they're thinking of you. You're ROB.* He's the most special man in the world to me — and not just to me. I know there are hundreds of folks out there for whom he has wrought miracles, who remember him years later for not just his skill as a physiotherapist, but his 'way' — Rob's way — which is unique, precious.

The updates serve multiple purposes. They create a web of love and support continually flowing back and forth. Over time, my BlackBerry gives me the ability to read the good wishes to Rob wherever we are — doctor's offices, chemotherapy, living-room.

For Rob, they create an energy flow directly to him. His response to the e-mails, the cards, is always one of amazement. Every flood of responses lifts him up, both physically and spiritually. Everybody is pulling for him.

Crucial for me, the updates also force me to look at the state of our lives in the moment. They keep me factual, instead of fast-forwarding into a time when there will be no need for updates. They keep me in the here and now, and sometimes, regardless of the fatality that looms, the here and now is good.

CHAPTER 5

The Heartline

⌒

Friday 4 September 2009
First Spiritual Care Session

Helen

I TAKE A DEEP BREATH. Initial visits are always rather like jumping off a cliff into the unknown and groundless, every single time. No matter how many people one sees in spiritual care, no matter how many times one connects with people in the most vulnerable and tragic moments of their lives, it always feels risky stepping into someone else's story, brand new, as the 'spiritual care provider.'

It's a loaded term. 'Spiritual,' what does that mean? It arouses suspicion almost universally. "Is she going to preach?" "Will she judge me?" "If I refuse to see her is God going to count that against me?" Nothing less than a complete self-offering — authentic, real, responsive, and *human* — will do.

As a spiritual care specialist in the London Regional Cancer Program I walk in many faith paradigms with people. Being utterly open to any and every possible path of the individual is fundamental. 'Spiritual care,' or authentic care for that matter, requires showing up, fully, without an agenda, even a subtle one, every single time. And, as for what 'worked' or 'helped' last time, one has to let it go and open and empty one's hands and heart to receive the new.

Aboriginal, Buddhist, Christian, and other wisdom paths have deeply influenced me, and I weave them together in my practice, trying to speak in language that communicates meaningfully with the person in front of me. Every day fellow human beings ask me to walk with them into the wilds of grief, death, despair, and heartbreaking loss. Living with deep roots of trust is the only way for me to sustain my own connections with life and prevent despair and grief at the sadness of it all from engulfing me. Every day the pain I encounter challenges those roots to grow deeper. And spiritual care is never a one-way street: the other person's story moves, challenges, and changes me.

As I leave my office to meet Rob and Jen, I know this young couple and their terribly difficult situation is going to challenge me to dig deep. As I walk up the stairs to the chemotherapy clinic, I am breathing, preparing. What will this initial visit bring? In our clinic I follow the chair numbers to find Jen and Rob from the daily list at the nursing station.

It is the darker and less attractive north end — 'depressing,' some patients call it. The chairs are close together, offering little privacy — certainly not a place I relish meeting people for the first time. Difficult for them to be free with their emotions and stories, difficult for me to assess their situation and core needs because of the lack of privacy.

I see Rob in the chemotherapy chair — a small, unassuming-looking man, his round face showing the familiar fatigue of most patients. His wife sits next to him. Jen is an attractive, well-groomed woman with a sadness as deep as the Grand Canyon etched in her face. Another woman is there, which makes my heart sink: an initial visit and assessment of the situation will be difficult, and my time is really tight today — the relentless reality of health care.

"Hi, I'm Helen from Spiritual Care." I introduce myself, looking at each of them, taking in their subtle responses. Introducing my role and garnering enough trust to continue has about a one-minute window. Being real and present is critical. Blow these moments, and you lose the right to stay in the room and in their process. Presence is medicine, and other people, in their raw and shattered states, feel its reality or its absence very quickly.

I continue, hoping to jog their memories about who I am, "Grace mentioned I'd be trying to meet you during this treatment, I think?"

I hope they remember. If people recall my name and who I am from the endorsement and referral, then there's a shred of trust already there. If they don't, then I usually have to de-escalate the horror of an unannounced visit from the 'spiritual person' and the fear of terrible news. Yet, in this case, the bad news was already the worst it could be.

'Oh, yes," Jen responds, with a slight flicker of positive recognition. "Helen, this is my boss, Donna. She's visiting with us."

"I can come back later, if you like." My gut tells me it's important to let them take the lead on their contact with me.

"No, it's OK," says Donna, "I'm leaving anyway. I'll leave you to visit."

I check out Jen's response.

"OK," she tells her friend. "See you later."

Inwardly I feel relief. I don't have to juggle my schedule.

I sit down.

What on earth could one possibly offer — short of a Lourdes miracle — that would mean anything to two people who are facing death, with young children, older children, and a recent marriage?

I lean into the old, familiar feeling of deep inadequacy that arises in the face of profound suffering and breathe, feet on the earth, as I've taught many, many people and learned long ago from my own teachers. Not for me to have the answers. Just be present. Stay open, follow the threads of their story, and allow inner, intuitive depths to guide us all.

Rob is looking at me, and I don't sense any aversion. Jen is sad and composed — rather like a glass that just one tap would shatter. I sense in her a despair because no one, including me, has anything to offer her. In a way, she's quite right. Myself is all I can offer — a hand in a wilderness in which I too am blind.

I introduce myself, offer a bit about who I am and what 'spiritual care' means. I let them know that I'm aware of the diagnosis and how sorry I am.

Jen begins to talk with fluidity, and a conversation evolves with relative ease. I am grateful. I listen with my body as much as my heart. I follow the subtle movements through my being as their story washes over me. I don't try to grab all the details — I absorb the tone, the feeling, the images. Usually when I stay present enough in a conversation a thread emerges that guides my instincts to follow it. It's rather like tracking a silent creature through the forest, letting it guide me slowly to the depths of the forest, where a kernel of 'something' lies. It takes an inner stillness, a lack of fear of the situation with the pain of it all, and, most of all, awareness in one's bones that death is never the last word about anything in life.

I listen to their narrative quietly.

Jen tells me how she and Rob met years before and eventually married. She describes experiencing for the first time what others meant by the phrase 'finding your soulmate' — a term she'd not really believed in before the moment she met Rob.

"It felt as if Rob and I had known each other before — perhaps many times before. And I don't believe that stuff really. But when we met, it was so powerful, so like nothing I've experienced before. I just *knew* him, and it felt like we'd been drawn together for a reason. We got married a couple of years later, and our love has just expanded ever since. It just got bigger and bigger. I would think, "How can I love him more?" But I would. Every day, it grew.

"Now ... " — the tears started rolling down her face. "Now, it's all being taken away. Pancreatic cancer is fatal. We know there is no cure. We're realistic."

She pauses. We sit in silence.

"We don't know how to do this," she adds.

I feel my own depths move with the sadness of it all. Yes, indeed, how on earth does one 'do' this?

Yet her sharing has been tweaking my attention. It is her use of the word 'soulmate.' A term I am more than familiar with, yet most of the time, when people say they've found their soulmate, I don't buy it at all. Time so often proves otherwise, and infatuation makes us hope against hope this is 'it.'

Yet something in their story, the energy underlying it and the energy present in the bond between them, is making me sit up and really believe Jen. It just feels authentic, and it is one of the first times I've actually felt this kind of authenticity in those words. It's tugging strongly on my awareness, a kind of magnetic pull of energy.

Jen has also revealed a shred of an innate spiritual value in her depths, albeit fragile and tentative. She has just unwittingly named an almost-inarticulate hope in the possibility that there is 'something' beyond her in this universe, an interconnection that drew them together. This sense of 'something' is coming from her experience of the synchronicities that crossed their paths, serendipitously at first, aligning things for their love to come into being. Here's the thread — the strength of love in their relation-ship and their experience of its mysterious emergence in their lives. Jen's own inner depths have revealed it.

I take up the thread and offer it back to them, giving it voice.

"Death may bring the end of a physical form of life, but it is not the death of a relationship." I pause to let the meaning of this notion sink in and to see how it lands. I see it catches their attention. There is a slight shift of energy, a deepening attentiveness, and they're both looking at me, very directly.

An old supervisor of mine used to say this, and I'd come, over the years, to see and experience the deep truth of it: relationship does not seem to 'end' with everyone when they pass through that veil we call 'death.' Many people over the years have told me stories of loved ones showing up, guid-ing, and speaking, in both their waking and their dream life. Far too many for me to dismiss this as 'mere imaginings.'

Years ago I'd read a book about a monk and a lay woman who inten-tionally strengthened their heart love for one another in preparation for his death so they could sustain their love and connection beyond it. She has spent the subsequent years sharing her story and the reality of his love that she still feels. An energetic partnership of love that stretches across the veil.

The book has lived like a seed in my mind all these years and right now comes back with force. It is possible. It can happen, perhaps, if the love is strong enough. It was for them. Maybe it will be for Jen and Rob. It's a thread, a small, invisible possibility.

"If you've been drawn together in this universe, as you believe," I con-tinue, "then Rob's death will not end this deep connection you have to one another energetically. Love doesn't 'end.' This," I pointed to my hand, "is energy."

Quantum physics has finally caught up with what Buddhists and many indigenous peoples have taught for millennia. The form dissolves, but the energy, love, does not disappear. It can't. We're in a closed system in this universe. Energy does not 'die.' It changes forms. When two people love each other deeply, they feel each other, even when they're not in the same room. That's the shared energy field. It perhaps does not simply evaporate when the body dies. It simply changes form.

I can feel Jen and Rob focusing intently on what I'm saying. My gut says I've found a hidden trail in the dark, dark forest.

I look at each of them and ask, "Do you find that you know how the other is when you're apart? That you think each other's thoughts?" I reach for their personal experience to ground what I'm saying. My hunch is that they would say "Yes." In the end, it's lived experience that creates trust. Not belief.

Jen nods, "Oh yes, always." Rob nods too. He has locked his eyes onto mine in such a magnetic way, it encourages me to keep going. Yet inwardly I am checking like crazy with my intuition to make sure this is so. It's not my practice to give homilies on energetics and to be actually offering a 'content' of 'hope' so quickly and with so little knowledge of the people's belief systems and experience. But something tells me we have little time here and this conversation is critical. Rob is gazing at me with an intensity that compels me to continue.

I take another deep breath from the depths and continue.

"Well, that's what I call 'the heartline.' It's the invisible thread between us that connects us. We are all one life form in this earth. It's a web of life, many forms, all one energy, and living, breathing energy. Essence remains beyond death; this is taught by many religious paths. Not all, but enough for me to believe they're pointing to something we can't grasp too easily. Your heartline is deep. That's clear. That won't break when Rob dies."

They're not resisting the truth of his diagnosis. I heard that very clearly in Jen's brief sharing of their situation. There is no appeal for cure here, and this is not a situation of having to silently hold onto reality in the face of deep resistance, as I often experience. They've gone there, accepted it, now they're asking about hope. What is hope in all this? Nothing less than something from the bones is going to cut it.

"So, how do we feel that?' asks Jen. "How does the heartline work?"

I hear in her question that this language, this new 'name' of 'something' that she's already experienced, has given Jen something to grab onto. There is a faint, faint trace of curiosity beneath the flatness of her despair. We don't grab onto what doesn't resonate. But this does. Sometimes we speak to the parts of people they're not yet even aware of, the aspects of themselves in their depths that have the inner strength and wisdom they need but that they have no idea how to connect with in the overwhelmingly bleak present moment.

"I have no expertise, just my intuition and limited experience myself with people who are both alive and also who have died," I answer, honestly. I don't tell them this is the first time I've ever spoken of the heartline to a couple in front of me, when one partner is dying. I'm embarking on a new trail here.

I share a couple of stories from my own recent experience. I sense again the intensity of Rob's attention. It's quiet and very, very present.

"I believe, if we are to accept some of the teachings, particularly from the Buddhists, that we can cultivate our inner awareness of the heartline and strengthen our energy body through meditation. The energy body lives on after the mortal body dies. We're all 'energy.' This is simply a way of speaking about the interconnectedness of all beings. It's believed that the masters, even those who have died, share their wisdom through transmission, through the heartline, energetically across time and space; a sort of 'download,' like we do from the internet, except this is a download from the web of life. It's believed the masters still transmit their wisdom, not dissimilar from the way Christians speak about Christ's guidance through his 'spirit.'"

I've no idea what Jen and Rob's childhood religious background is. I suspect their cradle experience was Christian, in some way, shape, or form. Sometimes it's helpful to thread together language from different religions to point to the intangible beyond the words.

I continue, "I believe we can cultivate this skill of connecting on the heartline. It's been lost to us in the scientific worldview that has prevailed for a few hundred years. But way too many people have told me stories about their experiences of their loved ones after they've died for me not to believe there's something to this. And our aboriginal peoples teach this wisdom too. They honour their ancestors, speak to them, hold feasts for them, and ask for their guidance. We, in Western society, are really the only society that doesn't really teach this."

I feel as if I am walking on a tightrope. I am tracking inwardly the thought that I am just trying to offer a band-aid of hope. Yet, as much as it startles me to realize where we're going, my gut says to trust it. I seem to be following something that is unspoken.

"How do we tell the kids?" Jen asks. "We've told Rob's children, Ben and Jessica. They are twenty-three and eighteen. My kids are only seven and eight. We haven't told them yet."

Yes, indeed. How? My own children's age. I notice the shift she's initiated back to the reality of their present moment.

"Tell them the truth," I respond. "Children will smell a withholding of truth from their parents a mile away. The unknown, what is kept from being in the room by the adults, is way scarier than the known and spoken. Tell them the truth, but that it's not now, Rob isn't dying right now, and there's a whole lot of living to do until he does die. Teach them that death is not the enemy, that it is part of life. Teach them it's OK to be sad, to cry, to weep together, and show them that you can still be in this together, that they are a part of this every step of the way. Bring them into it, don't shut them out.

"They're looking to you to teach them about this part of life. It's so soon, they're so young, and yes, it's really sad they now have to face losing their beloved step-dad to death as part of their life journey but it IS part of their life journey and they will get the PhD in how to truly live life from you in this process. They'll get what this world is not going to teach them and, in fact, what this world teaches them to fear terribly. Show them your grief, teach them that grief is OK, it's part of life, and you'll find life shows up in the midst of it all, and they'll learn that life never leaves them, even in the face of death."

I pause. I'm aware of how many words are spilling out. I feel the terrible sadness of it all, in them, in the air. Their eyes, however, have locked into mine. They're listening; they're not signalling me to stop — quite the opposite. I feel a silent urging to continue.

I dive in, following the inner currents moving in me. "Tough, tough path. Not one I'd wish on anyone. But here it is. You're on it, and this will shape their lives for the rest of their lives, and you can do the journey together. Teach them about the heartline, that Rob will be with them even after they can't see him. Teach them that this world is all one, that they can feel you and him when you're not with them. No school prepared you for this, but you're in the school of life now, and that means facing death in the eye and turning it into the teacher instead of the enemy. If your kids can get that through this journey with Rob held in your love, you've given them gold that is more valuable than anything any school can give them."

I can feel the energy between the three of us. It's an energy I know well from many sessions with people. It's the energy of having hit the mark, of speaking a language they understand, can grab onto. It's the energy of genuine hope arising.

Rob is nodding slightly. Jen finally says, "That's the first hopeful thing anyone has said to us. It's the first time I feel anything but devastated and shattered. Can we meet with you to practise this heartline thing?"

"Absolutely," I respond, more confidently than I feel. As much as I live this in my own life, experience it as very real, teach my own children the reality of the invisible energy of the universe (some might call it the 'god energy'), I have certainly never had sessions with patients to teach them this intentionally. I've just jumped into a potential professional suicide. If it doesn't happen, I've just set Jen up for the most spiritually devastating bereavement possible, if she doesn't feel anything of Rob after he's died. My intuition has taken me out on a huge limb here, and I am just hoping it is right.

Yet, with a deep breath, feet on the ground, I sense we're on the right path. 'Life' has happened here. Life has broken through a despair that was like a lead weight over their heads. Life has touched them with a stirring of hope, like a very subtle breeze. Again, 'something,' just like in Jen's story about their love emerging, something intangible, feels invisibly part of all this.

"When would you like to meet? Do you want to call and make a time?" I ask, leaving it as open-ended as possible. This is their process, and their timing needs to guide it.

"Yes, we'll call you when we have our schedule for the next few weeks,"

Jen says, and she adds: "Thank you so much for coming to see us. It's been really helpful."

Rob nods in agreement, again, with his steady gaze. "Thank you," he says.

I walk slowly back to my office. Something has happened here. There's a path we're all on together.

Friday 4 September 2009
The Drive Home

Jen

"WHAT DID YOU THINK OF HELEN?" I ask Rob as we make our way home from our first chemotherapy and meeting with Helen.

"She seems very nice," Rob replies. "What was that thing she said again? What did she call it?"

"The heartline?"

"Yes, I think we already have that," Rob states, as if it were an established fact.

"Do you think you'd want to go back and see her again?" I am going to run with anything that Rob thinks will help. Any thread or shred of possibility of hope is worth pursuing.

"Yes, definitely." Rob is not one to judge people quickly; he is very non-judgmental. One of the things I've loved about him always — there's always an open door, whoever you are, but he quickly decides whom he'll trust and keep going with and whom he won't. He would keep supporting patients long after other people gave up; he was known for his persistence and faith in people's ability to improve from strokes and health problems.

But I know Rob wouldn't entertain more of this spiritual-care stuff if he wasn't completely into it. Time is too short. Life is too precious to waste any energy. His 'Yes' is emphatic and clear. Whoever Helen is, whatever she has to offer, he is in. Which means so am I.

"Well, we'll have to see how you are after chemotherapy, and we can probably schedule it when you have your next chemotherapy so we don't have to do two drives in." We live almost an hour out of London, and it

is a lot for Rob to drive into the city and takes precious energy from him.
"Yes," he says.

He's clear. And so am I. This heartline thing, this notion of our deep
connection being something that we can focus on for our time together
that's left, this is a sliver of something no one else has given us so far — a
shred of focus, a scrap of hope. It gives us something more than counting
days as we have begun to do.

Thursday 10 September 2009
Rob Update

We're heading back into round two of chemotherapy tomorrow, thought
we'd give you an update. Feel free to pass on. Rob came through the first
round of chemotherapy very well, not too many side effects, a couple of
days of feeling like he had the flu. Nausea was intermittent but well controlled with a super-duper anti-emetic for chemotherapy patients.

Rob's pain is well controlled, needing only minimal breakthrough drugs
throughout the day and night (breakthrough drugs are "extra" doses on
top of his baseline dose of pain drugs that he takes when his pain "breaks
through"). We're hopeful that the chemotherapy may further reduce pain
and the need for narcotic pain management.

Energy is pretty low, lots of rests throughout the day, and little or no
energy for activities. This is of course a big shift as you know Rob is typi-
cally pretty go, go, go. We did get to Waterloo on Wednesday to visit Jessica in her university residence. I moved her in on Labour Day as Rob wasn't
up to it only three days after chemotherapy so Rob and I went up for a
brief visit so he could see where she lives. He was exhausted afterwards
but glad we did it. We'll try and go back again in the next couple of weeks.

We so appreciate the outpouring of support from everyone. The most
energetic I see Rob get every day is when we walk to the post office to
check the mail. It's very English I think, this preoccupation with the post
but Rob loves getting the get-well cards people have been sending. Word
has reached far and wide of his illness. So many old acquaintances are
sending their best wishes, which Rob loves. So please anyone who reads

this; keep sending mail. Thanks also to everyone who sent various food parcels; that has been a huge help to me.

Rob's twin brother Malcolm and his wife Caroline are arriving on Saturday and staying for a week. Rob is looking forward to seeing them, as am I.

Sunday 20 September 2009
Rob Update

Rob has completed his third treatment of this first chemotherapy round this past Friday September 18th. Chemotherapy itself went fine. Rob had a rough day on Saturday, but his biggest complaint is significant fatigue, and general "under the weather" type feeling. By Sunday afternoon, he was beginning to pick up a bit so this is doable.

We now have a week off, and start chemotherapy again on Monday Sept 28th. We see the oncologist that day as well to discuss how Rob has tolerated the chemotherapy. We are going to try and get away to Niagara on the Lake with Rob's son Ben during the week off if Rob feels up to it, something we had promised Ben earlier in the summer prior to Rob's diagnosis.

Rob's twin brother Malcolm left after a week's visit on Saturday September 19th. They played golf once, and got to the driving range another time. It was a nice visit, a hard goodbye.

We have continued to receive many cards, e-mails, and messages of good will. I am typing this e-mail from our computer in our dining room. Our dining room table is almost filled with cards, and the side-board is full. I often come in here and read them when Rob is sleeping. These incredible messages, hopes and prayers have given both of us so much strength. Thanks to everyone who has sent thoughts our way.

He looks good, drinking tea as I write this, still positive and funny. What else would any of us expect!

Part Two

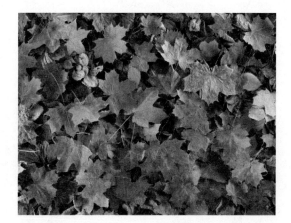

Autumn 2009

Chapter 6

A Path Opens

∞

Jen

I AM SITTING AT the computer and looking around at all the cards on our table from our friends and well-wishers. An outpouring of care that is amazing to receive. I am looking at them all. I feel so very lost. Many are sympathy cards. I am thinking to myself, *I really need to call Helen. I don't know how to do this. How are we going to do this?*

The phone rings. "Hi, Jen, it's Helen, I was wondering how you're doing since we talked?"

"This is so weird," I respond. "I was just thinking I was going to call you. I am sitting looking at all these cards people have sent us." This is uncanny. "The chemotherapy has gone OK," I continue. "We've had one round of chemotherapy, and he's doing OK. It hasn't hit him as badly as we'd thought. I can't believe how many cards have come. We walk to the post office every day, Rob has energy to just get there and back, and he really looks forward to the cards. They've been amazing what people have written."

We talk for a while, and Helen asks if we want to come back for more time together. I say yes. Rob has grabbed onto this, and so have I.

Helen has an opening before Rob's next chemotherapy, so I book us in. Again, another moment of good timing.

Friday 2 October 2009
Second Spiritual Care Session

Jen

IT SEEMS A LONG TIME since we've seen Helen. A lot has happened, and Rob is sick; we aren't yet seeing benefits of chemotherapy, only side effects. I am hoping Helen can help us in some way, I have no idea how.

I am not focusing on anything other than how we can do this. I have in my mind that we'll make it to Christmas, but I haven't thought much beyond that. We have only a short time to figure out all this spiritual stuff, what it's all about for us. I have no idea what Rob really wants from this. I feel I have a better sense of Helen because Rob was so tired and drugged when we met her, but I know he really wants to see her again.

It surprises me so much to be in contact with spiritual care and how we've managed to connect. I wonder if only people who are dying receive referral to spiritual care. What does it all mean? I have no idea where Helen fits into the cancer program and whom she normally sees.

We feel anxiety heading into chemotherapy. Will Rob's blood work be OK? Will he be able to have the treatment? It is always dodgy, and so much is riding on his having it — time is so, so short. We're buying it in hours and days with every session.

We reach Helen's door and knock. She is on the phone and beckons us in.

I look around the room, and it is unlike any other office in the hospital I've ever seen. There's a couch with knitted shawls on the arms, probably knit by some person with cancer, I think. There are rocks and seashells, bits of grass. An interesting picture of a colourful ... ? What? Something on the wall. What kind of place is this?

I also notice pictures of her children on the wall, and I see they're the same age as Jack and Haley. That reassures me — she's a mother, she gets that part. I am trying to figure out her religious background from the clues in her room. She mentioned Buddhism and Christianity and native traditions when we met. Who knows?

I look at Rob. He's taking this all in as well, calmly, without judgment, as always. I wonder how his energy is going to be.

Helen greets us warmly and hugs us both — heartfelt. We sit down.

She asks about the treatments, how they're going, and what our treatment schedule is, and then, after we've explained that, she asks more slowly, "How *are* you?"

"Not too bad," Rob replies briefly. "Doing all right."

Helen explains to him that she and I talked on the phone last week: "It sounds like you've had a busy month."

"Yes," he explains. "Since you met us before, I've had a round of chemotherapy, seen the oncologist, met with our nurse practitioner, Grace, and the palliative care physician has been out to our house a couple of times. We're going to continue with chemotherapy. It's not as bad as I expected."

"You still have your hair!" Helen comments with a smile.

"Yes, I still haven't lost my hair!" Rob responds, with a slight grin.

I add, "Pain is much better controlled since last time, we're getting on top of that, and now we're just working on managing side effects."

I wonder how much medical stuff Helen wants or needs to know. I'm reading up on pancreatic cancer, rapidly becoming an expert on every possible aspect that I can understand. I am also studying every bit of research I can get my hands on about the drugs he's taking.

But how to live all this with this inevitable fatality knocking on our door? How do we *live?* That I can't seem to find any answers for.

"We told the little ones." Rob says, referring to Jack and Haley. "We already told Ben and Jessica right after the diagnosis back in August, but Jessica was in the room when we told Jack and Haley."

"How did that go?" Helen asks, gently. I can feel the care in her voice.

"It was very hard, probably one of the hardest days in my life," Rob continues.

Tears prick my eyes as he tells Helen about one of the most harrowing experiences of my life — telling my young children that their beloved Rob, their step-dad, was going to be dying. We had learned it could be only weeks away. We didn't have the luxury of keeping it from them or waiting for a 'better time.' There might not be more time.

I continue. "We told them on Labour Day weekend, the Saturday before they started back to school, right after we saw you last, Helen. We sat them down and said, 'We have some difficult news. You know Rob hasn't been well? We've found out from the doctors that Rob has cancer.'

"Haley burst into tears and asked Rob, 'Are you going to die?' Rob said, 'Yes, but not right away.' Haley asked, 'Can't the doctors do anything?' Rob said, 'Yes, they're giving me lots of medicine so that I don't die right away.'"

I'm finding this so difficult to talk about. Helen is really listening and looks moved. I look at Rob, and he's staring right at me and holds my hand.

I go on. "Then Rob said to them, 'And when I die, I'll always be with you, I'll find a way to help you. I'll be right there in the classroom listening to what your teachers are teaching you. You can *always* talk to me; I'll hear you, and I'll be there.' Haley asked, 'Well, how can we talk to you when you're dead?' Rob replied, 'Well, my body will be dead, but my spirit will be alive.'"

I continue the story. "Haley clung to me, crying; she hugged Rob. Jessica was crying on the couch, a few feet away. We had told her a few weeks before, as soon as Rob was diagnosed. Jack refused to be held, tears were streaming down his face. Finally, a few minutes later, he let himself be hugged. Slowly everyone left. It was awful."

I can see Helen taking all this in. I can see how moved Rob is reliving this story with me. "It was so hard." The memory is flooding me. I go on, "Haley came back into the room a little while later where we were sitting just numb from it all. 'Robbie, were you sad when the doctor told you that you had cancer?' she asked. Rob said, 'Yes, I am sad. It's very sad.'"

Helen is silently nodding. She has tears in her eyes, which surprises me. Surely she hears stories like this day in and day out?

"Well, bravo for speaking the truth to them," she says. "So hard to do. What children imagine is so much worse than what they are told truthfully and directly. You told them it won't be right away, you've brought them into the process alongside you, not shut them out.

"Anxiety rises acutely," she adds, "when kids feel something is being withheld. They can feel it in the air, the awfulness of it. That is scarier than parents speaking to them directly, bringing them *into* the experience with them where they are. At least they are connected instead of disconnected.

"You did a brave, brave thing. You didn't shy away from the truth of it. Now they get to live *with* you in this, alongside you, be a part of it all. You gave them a great gift. As painful as it is."

I hear Helen, but it was so awful, her words don't make it any less painful.

I continue. "It's really hard to talk to children about death when they are children who are so concrete and think very concretely. Your job as a parent is to protect your children. I certainly didn't feel like I was protecting them by telling them Rob was dying. We can't protect them from this."

"Nature is your best teacher for the children," Helen responds. "For all of us, really. If you look at death in nature, it's always part of a cycle. When does a tree die? It falls, goes to the earth, and becomes soil. Things grow in that soil, a 'dead' tree has all kinds of life growing out of it. Kids relate to the cycles in nature. They get it. You can turn them to nature to show how things die and change forms but the life process, the essence, remains, always changing but always remaining and evolving. Nature is our best teacher and our best healer for scared and broken hearts."

I think, *OK, Helen, I'll try it.* I am so at sea; I have no idea how we are going to do this. I'll run with anything that makes the remotest sense. This has a shred of sense in it. "We'll see if the nature thing works," I say. I don't feel an aversion to what she is saying, but I have no idea if it will be at all helpful. I trust that she must have lots of experience with helping families with children, and she has her own. That is enough for me to trust and try it.

Helen asks about Rob's family in England. Since our last session with her, Rob's parents, Malcolm and his wife, Caroline, and their younger brother, Howard, and his wife, Lynn, have all been over from England. We are gearing up for another visit from his parents and also his best friend from high school. It has been so busy. As a result of telling Rob's family the prognosis, everyone immediately came to see us.

"We have so little time," I say again. "We have been told to expect weeks to months. Twelve more weeks would get us to Christmas."

Reaching Christmas is what we had asked — begged for — when we met with the oncologist. We know the reality that Rob will die soon. I just really hope Helen can help us find the best possible way to live this time that remains. I know a cure isn't on the cards. So does Rob.

"Neither of us is wasting any time or energy wishing for what is outside the realm of 'likely,'" I add.

It also isn't just Christmas. I know if we can reach that, then we'll have made it to all the children's birthdays and my own, as well as our third wedding anniversary. We will have celebrated all the big events – except Rob's birthday — if we can make it to December 25. I am hoping against hope that we'll have that time. It's my hourly cry, my prayer: "More time. Please, get us to Christmas."

Helen asks, "So, what is hope in this moment? What do you hope for?"

"I hope for time," I respond quickly. Ever since the diagnosis, time is all I've asked for. "I am so afraid this cancer is going to eat Rob alive. When he was first diagnosed and we were told weeks, I didn't know then that we'd make it to this day. At least we're still here. I just want time."

"You're in a really tough moment. Cure is not on the table, and you're being very courageous by facing that truth, not clinging to what is most unlikely. I find it more helpful, for anyone, even those without cancer, to focus on 'How do I want to live right now, today, this moment, tomorrow?' rather than focusing on a future we can't control or manipulate.

"You are on the crash course in living in the present moment, but this requires facing the pain of the present as well as seeking the gifts of being in the 'now.' We often mentally run to an impossible future or cling to the longed-for past because right now is just so terribly painful. You're choosing to stay right here, in the pain of facing Rob's mortality.

"And you're asking so courageously the critical question, 'How do we do this?' It's the Zen koan of cancer, of life really: 'How do I live when I know I am dying?' There are many teachers across the ages who have offered that embracing the reality of death, right here, right now, is the way to begin truly living.

"What hope means, in this conundrum, is for each of us to work out. And that's what I hear so much that you've both set your face to. Squarely. And it is work. It doesn't come easily or cheaply. It means grappling with the pain of it all, the fears, the unknown, which you're both so very bravely doing."

There is something that happens when Helen talks, a comforting sense of her wrapping us in care, that makes us believe that somehow, some way, we'll get through this. It is like a sense of integrating instead of disintegrating, albeit fleeting.

"You have an amazing relationship that I can see; I feel it between you. Your love is very authentic and deep. This is your great gift, and that's not going to get shattered or taken away by death. This is what you can teach your children. They are silently watching, looking to you as their elders for how to face death, look it in the eye and take a hold of life with two hands, and truly live each and every moment until that last breath."

I am taking all of this in. I wonder how Rob is doing, sitting next to me on the couch. Is this hitting the mark for him? I sense that it is. Even though Helen is speaking about death and 'last breaths,' she's not talking about survival statistics, and that is a refreshing change.

She continues, "You have your love, you have your deep soul connection and bond, and you can show your children that this is what life is about. Love, connection, togetherness, and community in the face of struggle. You can reach your hand out to your children and draw them into that love and show them that living doesn't mean pretending death doesn't exist. It means facing death squarely and using it as a portal to dive through into living, into loving each other, right now in this moment.

"You're choosing a courageous path by not clinging to the less-than-one-per-cent possible miracle that almost no one with pancreatic cancer gets to experience, if ever. You're choosing to face it head on, and you have the chance to discover something powerful, something your children will absorb by osmosis and draw on when they face their own crossroads and suffering down the road in their lives."

Helen pauses, and there is a moment of silence as we absorb not just the words but also the feeling that is happening between and behind the words.

Then she quietly adds, "At the end of sessions, I often end with meditation. Would you like to explore some meditation that you can work with together at home?"

This suggestion rather startles me and makes me uncomfortable. I look around the room again and see the shells, the picture, and the rocks, and suddenly I wonder where we are and what this is all about. I feel very uncomfortable.

I look at Rob for his reaction, and he seems very calm and not at all surprised. I dive in, for his sake. If he's OK with this, it can't harm us to try it.

"So, let's close our eyes, and I'd like to suggest that you don't hold hands," Helen begins.

This idea rather upsets me. We always hold hands; we are always connected in some way.

Helen explains, "I'd like to take you through a practice to become more aware of your own energy and each other's, and it's easier to cultivate that energetic awareness if you're not touching by holding hands."

I release Rob's hand, rather reluctantly.

She goes on, "Become aware of your breath. Feel the rhythm of your breathing: the inhale, the exhale, the pause between them. Become aware of your feet, take in the breath, and feel life flowing into your body; breath is life, life is breath. Feel the releasing of life, of the breath — we cannot hold onto it, we cannot cling, and our bodies have this truth embedded right into our breathing."

Her voice is very calming; I can feel myself relaxing into the words, into my breath. I can feel Rob beside me, very calm.

"Now, notice your energy, feel your own presence. Feel your body and the space that it occupies in space and time. Feel where you meet the couch, the ground. Let your whole body feel — our minds so often are the busy world we live in. But our bodies are feeling so much all the time, so aware of many dimensions, sensations of what is around us.

"Drop into your body awareness. Let your body 'aware' itself. Now, with your inner eye, see inwardly your body-presence. Notice your own presence, which is energy, quantum physics tells us that.

"Is there a colour that you see as you inwardly look at your own body from within? Allow the image of your own inner presence; your own energy field arises into your awareness. Trust what comes.

"Now concentrate on each other. Can you sense where the other is? What is their energy, what does it look like, feel like? What quality of energy is their body-presence? Notice what you notice without judgment or censoring, just trust what you feel. Feel into each other's presence from within, with your inner awareness.

"Notice how you can feel where you are and where they are. Now notice that you can feel the shared field of awareness that you are, that you are connected. Can you tell where you end and they begin? Is there an ending or beginning, or a shared experience of flow between you?

"In truth, we are all one vast web of energy, differing forms, but profoundly interconnected in this web of life we call the earth. Feel into this experientially with your awareness of each other right here, feel your shared field of presence, the oneness that you are in essence."

I am noticing that I can really feel what she is saying. I am in a whole new world, or a whole new world has just opened up, and I've dived into it. It's so real and also very strange. I am no longer uncomfortable. This is so … something I can't even put words to.

Helen continues, "Now, with this inner awareness, feel right *into* each other's energy and presence. See if you can feel each other, from within one another's energy, from the inside, as if you're right inside them."

I notice that the room has become utterly still. Everything feels silent and full of nothing but Helen's voice and our presence with one another.

I suddenly notice that I can feel Rob. Feel his energy, different from mine, but connected. I can feel his pain in his body in my own solar plexus, where his pancreas is — it is like a shelf in my belly. I can feel a dizziness that is almost disconcerting because it is so strong. I can feel Rob feeling into me, I can feel him *inside* my own energy or body, or I'm not sure how I am feeling him but know that I am.

I wonder if I am experiencing his body experience of being on the strong drugs, the dizziness — the room is spinning and feeling slightly out of my body. I can see a yellowish-white colour in a ball of light that is like the sun, and I know it is Rob. There is black all around it, with this glowing, warm light, pulsing, moving, radiating into the blackness around it. I am seeing Rob from within.

I lose myself in the experience and feel total connection to it in amazement. Then my mind jumps in, *What is this? What is Rob experiencing?* Then the energy and Helen's voice take me back into the feeling in my abdomen, which is unfamiliar, and the discomfort that I am sure is Rob's pain. *Is this for real? Am I really feeling this? Is this really Rob? Is this actually possible?* I want to believe it is.

I feel almost nauseous it is so real. I am hot. Some part of me feels a truth to this experience. My gut is feeling that this is very real. It is an incredible feeling of connection. It's startling — like seeing someone I love for the first time after being absent for a while. I am finding Rob from within, in an intangible world I've touched before. My mind keeps jumping in and questioning, I can't stay with it, but something keeps drawing me back. It's as real as day.

It reminds me of the very first time Rob and I held hands. When he first touched my hand saying goodbye, a bolt of hot energy ran through my body. It jolted me and awakened an instant connection of deep love. It was the moment that marked the beginning of our love, which has kept expanding through the years into something so profound that the word 'love' barely captures it.

Now, facing his dying, meditating in this woman's office, I am having a similar experience. The deep connection between us, now taking another dive deeper, into death, but also, in this moment, something that feels beyond death. More real than his body, more real than mine.

This is a world Rob is more familiar with. He would never say in his work that he and the patient were going to do a visualization. He'd say, "OK, Mrs. Smith, you're going to imagine rocking forward in the chair and what your feet will feel like on the floor. Imagine straightening your spine, taking a big breath, and feeling 'Of course, I can walk.'"

If it was someone with a problem in their hand, he'd say, "I want you to imagine all those bones and muscles moving together. They know exactly what to do, and they're all going to move together and pick up this coffee cup, because your muscles know what to do."

Rob would say all the time, "Muscles have memory." This came from a physiotherapy technique that he had trained in and used extensively. He, as usual, had adapted it in his 'Rob way' into special ways of doing things. People would start walking who weren't supposed to walk, and he believed in people until they believed in themselves.

Sitting in Helen's office, following her meditations, for Rob it draws on a part of himself that he's used professionally with his own patients. Now she's helping him to draw on it in the face of his own dying. He knows this world much better than I.

Now I know what he has been talking about. This feels more real than 'hope.' This gives me something to walk away with that no one can take away. I don't care what we call it. For the first time, I feel something beyond the terrible grief of losing him. I've *felt* him, in his essence, and that gives me a feeling of something I've not felt since the diagnosis; something beyond hope, a sense of the 'real' that somehow death cannot annihilate.

Helen brings us gently back into the room and asks us what our experience was.

"Rob, did you feel Jen's energy?"

"Oh, yes, very much."

It thrills me to hear him say this. So he had felt it too, like I did.

"What was it like?" Helen asks him.

"Yellow light." Same as I!

"What else did you feel in Jen?"

"I also felt her concern and her worry for me." He adds, "And I felt her love."

I jump in. Helen asked Rob first, and his experience is so similar to mine. It's uncanny. We both saw yellow light.

"That was incredible," I add. "I felt a pressure in my abdomen like a shelf, like it was his pain. It was amazing." I feel the tears running down my face. "It's like nothing I've ever experienced before except when he first held my hand."

I am wondering how Helen does this.

Then I notice the time. It's time for chemotherapy. Helen also notices the clock.

"So, this can be your practice," she continues. "What you felt is the love you've had between you over the years. This is your connection, your heartline. Practise this when you're going to sleep, when you're in the house. Jen, when you're in the kitchen and Rob is in another room. This is the heartline, the energetic connection we all share. With practice it can be strengthened.

"It's not unreasonable to think that this bond can transcend death. Many spiritual traditions have pointed to this in different ways. That this connection between you is larger together than it is individually, and this bond of love you've cultivated surrounds your family, your children, and they're a part of it. Remember that energy in the universe is a closed system, it just goes on and on, changing forms perhaps, but never disappears.

It won't disappear after Rob's death."

Now, I am fully present with this idea. I have grabbed on because I've experienced this moment today. I truly believe it. Rob and I have a deep connection. I can hold onto that and focus on it, right here, right now, every day.

Helen asks, "If you'd like to come back again, you can call me."

"We'll definitely come back." Rob says. I look at him, noticing his emphatic decision.

We're coming back. A path has opened.

"Call me when it suits you. All the best with chemotherapy," Helen says. We hug. "Goodbye."

We walk out of Helen's office. It is a stark change to walk out of that cocoon into the busy corridors and clinic areas.

"We have to do lots of this, Rob," I say. I don't want to lose this experience. I don't want to lose Rob.

"We will," Rob says.

We walk to chemotherapy.

Saturday 3 October 2009

Jen

I HELP ROB upstairs to bed for his afternoon nap. The chemotherapy effects are making him feel quite unwell.

"I keep thinking of our session with Helen yesterday," I comment. "Did you really feel all that stuff? I keep wondering if I'm imagining what I felt." I feel a pressure to keep this conversation short because I know Rob needs his rest, but I ask anyway. I need to know.

Rob responds, "Yes, it happened. You were a yellow light."

I say, "Rob, I really hope I can still feel this when you're gone."

"I'm not going anywhere. I'm right here," he answers.

He tries to make himself comfortable in the bed.

"Well, you've made it to Haley's birthday," I say, with some amazement. It's today. She's at her Dad's place -- we've rescheduled our weekends so that after Rob's chemotherapy the kids are with their father. Rob has a quiet weekend to recuperate.

Rob smiles, "Yup, I made it." There is a pause.

"You have a birthday coming up too, I'm going to have to go shopping," he says, with a hint of sadness in his voice, because shopping would be hard for him right now.

I reply, "Write me a letter. I don't want anything from the store. Just write me a letter."

Thursday 8 October 2009
Birthday Letter from Rob to Jen

For Jen

This birthday wish comes from my heart. As we travel our path of life together through troubled times and happy moments, I always remember your smile and my love for you.

We can now spend all of every day together instead of snapshots during each day. Our paths are intertwined for a reason as they became many years ago although we did not know why.

I look forward to all of our tomorrows and enjoying all of our todays whilst savouring our yesterdays. We have many special moments still to make and experience and I look forward to making them with you from this day onwards.

I feel we have connections beyond what anyone could ever explain. Our soul connections or heartlines which drew us together and hold us together are stronger with each passing day and we will have all of our connections far beyond our life and lives.

I believe in us and will continue forever to love you and share my feelings, my heart and soul with you.

All my love
Forever
Rob

Mid-October 2009

Jen

WE'RE SITTING on the couch in the living-room. Jack and Haley launched their school year weeks ago. We have delivered Jessica to residence, and she has started university. Ben is working. We are in a lull of a few days between visitors from overseas. We've had a round of chemotherapy treatments. It is October. Autumn.

Our days are quieter now. A rhythm is quietly emerging. Rob's days are very routine, with regular medication, small, simple meals that his system can manage, and afternoon naps. His symptoms are so much better if he stays in a routine. Through trial and error over the past five weeks I have figured out what combination of daily events works best — no small task. I am so grateful for my previous work experience in health care. Of course we have so many appointments with doctors, nurses, chemotherapy, clinics, but I am trying so hard to keep the days in between calm.

We talk all day, every day. We talk about when we were young, the early days of each of our children's lives, Rob's hopes for their futures. We talk about our past five years together and how wonderful they have been. We talk about the inevitability of the end. We talk about him a lot. How is his pain, his nausea, his appetite, and so on, and so on? My constantly asking him how he's doing must wear him out. Very Rob, he responds often, "At this very second, I am feeling all right."

"So how are you doing, Rob?" I inquire for the three hundredth time today.

"I'm doing all right," he says. So calm. I notice he looks reflective.

"Whatchya thinking, sweetheart?" I ask. Another question that Rob hears all day, every day, from me. I know some day soon I won't be able to ask him. These conversations are like putting money in the bank. I don't know how many more weeks I'll be able to hear his voice.

"I think the golf balls are doing all right," he states, as if we were talking about golf balls just yesterday.

"What golf balls?" I ask. I'm lost. Two minutes ago we were talking about the English football (soccer) league. Now golf?

"My red golf balls. In my pancreas and my liver?" he queries with a smirk, as if I had momentarily forgotten that he had terminal metastatic cancer.

"Oh. Those golf balls," I say, smiling. "Well, what's going on with them these days?" I figure I'll go along with this game; Rob seems to be enjoying it enormously.

"Well, I sort of imagine the chemotherapy going in there and attacking the golf balls; sort of chipping the outside away. Then the Roombas come along and clean up the debris." He has a big smile on his face as he looks at my puzzlement.

"And Rob, what exactly is a Roomba?" I ask, baffled, truly wondering if I had perhaps given him the wrong dose of his powerful pain medication earlier.

"You know Roombas, those robot vacuums that suck up all the dirt on the floor. They're like a circular disc, and they bump into walls and then go back into the middle of the room and keep sucking up the dirt when you go away to work for the day. I'll show you one on the internet." He's gesturing wildly in front of his abdomen as he describes this imaginary robotic wonder.

"So how big is your Roomba?"

"Oh, just little," he explains, "so it can zoom around my pancreas and my liver." He says this so matter-of-factly. He's still grinning.

"Well," I ask with raised eyebrows, "is it working?"

"Yes, I think it is," he says. I sniff a little hope here.

"Well, then maybe you should spend some time every day putting it to work. Spend some time when you're drifting off for your nap imagining the chemotherapy and those Roombas disintegrating your golf balls. I don't think it can hurt?" I say.

I figure at any moment the degree-granting institution that bestowed my bachelor of science on me is going to leap out and take it away. What were we talking about here? It doesn't matter. Rob is lively and cares deeply about this story, and therefore so do I. This is the first time he has mentioned anything about his interacting with this thing that is taking over his body.

"Yes, ma'am," he says, smiling.

Thursday 22 October 2009
Our Wedding Anniversary

Jen

TODAY IS OUR THIRD anniversary. Rob's friend Dave is visiting from England and staying in Jessica's room. Rob's parents are here from England too, and they're in the guest room. We have a full house.

It's been such a full day. Lots of distractions have helped me forget for moments that this is our last anniversary together. I have to tell somebody about today.

Grace and I have exchanged many clinical e-mails. A level of trust and closeness has developed between Rob and Grace and me, and visits in our living-room probably strengthen it. Today I feel that I want to include her in this very non-clinical way.

Thursday 22 October 2009
E-mail from Jen to Grace

> *Grace,*
>
> *I had to share this with you. Got too distracted on Wednesday with other topics to tell you about Tuesday, but wanted to share and show you a couple of pictures.*
>
> *On Tuesday, I had a call from one of our Norwich neighbours that Rob has gotten to know over the past few years. His name is Darryl; he's a business man, lovely man, but more importantly he's involved in the local car club. People who know Rob know how much he loves old British sports cars. Well, Darryl had heard about Rob. In fact, we often see Darryl at the Cancer Clinic with his wife who is going through cancer treatment as well.*
>
> *Anyway, Darryl called me Tuesday morning. He was just getting ready to put his British racing green, nineteen-seventy-two TR6 away for the winter, and wondered if Rob would like to borrow it for the day. Rob's friend Dave owned Triumphs in his youth in England,*

and was so excited.
   I told Rob when he woke up and what a spring in his step. (So as I write this I'm not sure if it was the car or the deximethazone that caused the health turnaround?) I've attached a couple of pictures. The guys took the car out for a drive through the countryside and then Rob took me out for a spin as well. Fantastic, a bucket list moment for sure!
   Talk soon
   Jen

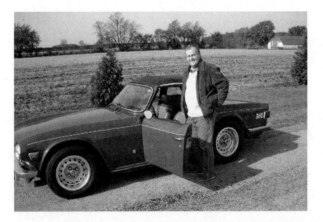

Sending a personal e-mail to Grace is provoking me to reflect on the impact she's had on us, and in such a short time. My work hat kicks in, and the people who are in charge of securing funding for nurse practitioners in the community need to hear about this.

It's late, but I fire off an e-mail to Donna, my boss and also Grace's.

Thursday 22 October 2009
E-mail from Jen to Donna (Jen's boss)

   Hi Donna,
   This is great news about the LHIN [Local Health Integration Network] wanting to profile nurse practitioners in the community, and I think it would be great if our experience with Grace could be

used to somehow make a case for the exceptional role the nurse practitioner plays. If you want to identify me and Rob, that is FINE with
me too. I give you express permission to use our names and if you
don't that's fine too. Maybe having a face to put to a name would help,
maybe not.

Grace has made such a tremendous difference to us. Remember,
how I told you about my "system navigation" dream that I had not long
after Rob was diagnosed? The one with all the stairs that I am carrying
him up and down and finally the doctor says, "I can't do anything for
your husband." I've often thought that at some time in my future I will
use this in a talk, but I can't imagine having the strength to say it out
loud without tears. I had it two days after Rob was diagnosed.

I take from the dream that the incredible sea of barracudas and
impossible challenges that I felt I was facing in the beginning — drugs,
chemotherapy, treatment options and lack of them, pain management,
C.T. results, biopsy results, sleep deprivation, GRIEF — I felt that it
ALL fell on me and I needed to get Rob through it and I could, but it
was terribly difficult.

And I guess all I can say is that I do not feel that way now that I
have Grace. She never says "there is nothing we can do"; even though
I know there is nothing that will cure Rob's cancer. She always solves
the little problems that present themselves every day times ten. I
ALWAYS feel better and more in control after I have spoken to her or
had a visit with her. I guarantee she has no idea what an impact she
has made in both of our lives. I truly feel that without her constant
steady, calm, positive but realistic way, I would not be able to cope in
this most unbelievably impossible situation I find myself in. The first
time she ever came, she asked not about Rob's health, but about our
kids and how they were handling things, she gets it.

Anyway, it's very late and I need to get off to bed. Hopefully some
of this can help.

Thanks for the good wishes. Some time we need to meet up again
for a glass of wine and a good chat.

Talk soon

Jen

CHAPTER 7

What Will Death Look Like?

◌◌

Tuesday 17 November 2009
Home Visit from Grace

Jen

ROB HAS BEEN PUT on steroids for quite a while, and this can contribute to adrenal insufficiency. I am aware that he needs to somehow reduce the steroids, and Grace is here for another bi-weekly check-in.

We are approaching Christmas, and it may be the end. The cancer is probably going to take over. Grace spends the first forty-five minutes looking at Rob's symptoms and all his medications. She's searching for what kind of tweaking of the meds needs to happen.

Today, as I watch her assess Rob, it strikes me anew how much she impresses me. Her clinical skills are astounding. She picks up on subtle changes with amazing clarity and accuracy and always seems to have a trick up her sleeve for treating Rob's symptoms.

I have always been someone who respects a good mind, a big brain, but there's more than just this with Grace. There is never pity, never any of the artificial sweetness that we have both encountered in health care. Grace is very genuine. I know in my bones that she cares about Rob, about both of us.

I wonder how she's developed this level of skill. She has mentioned that she comes from a big family. She has told me she is the youngest. She grew up on a farm and has clearly worked hard all her life, and the "make do" attitude that often accompanies a farming upbringing comes across in how she practises. She just makes it work. Thank goodness we have her.

Today, as I look at Rob, he is so sick. I can see it in his face and body as we sit in our living-room with Grace.

As her assessment comes to an end, we discuss the pros and cons of having the CT scan that's on for next week. Grace is weighing them all with us: "Knowing the results may take the wind out of your sails if it's showing progression. If it's showing regression or stability, then there's affirmation in continuing your course of treatment. It's totally your decision.

"Some people can't live without the concrete data. Some people can't live with it. The results won't influence your treatment at this point. The chemotherapy will continue because there's always the question of if he's not on the chemotherapy imagine how quickly it would have grown. So continuing will be the course of action. It's more about knowing what's happening and whether you think that's necessary."

"I want to know," insists Rob.

Whatever Rob says. It's his call. His life.

There is a pause.

Rob asks, "Can you tell us what to expect?"

"What do you mean, Rob?" Grace queries.

"How will this all end?"

I can't believe he's asking this. I look at him and think, "Are you really asking this?" Tears well up in me. I can't believe we're about to have this conversation.

Grace takes a deep breath and sits back in her chair. Up till now she has been her usual pragmatic self, sitting forward, solving problems, adjusting medications, and now she shifts gears.

"I am taking my oncology hat off and putting my palliative hat on," she says, always clear, always direct.

This conversation has long terrified me. But I know he's asking this for me. I need to know this. I need to prepare.

"Well, at the Community Care Access Centre we have a program called 'Expected Death in the Home.' Rob, you've told me before that your wish would be to die here at home. Expected Death in the Home involves a cascade of paperwork. Normally there is a team of nurses in the home who are part of the care, and the paperwork is set up in advance to prepare for this.

"When you actually die, if the nurse isn't already here, she'll be called. She'll come and do the pronouncement. Nurses are allowed now to do this — the coroner no longer needs to be called, and no ambulance needs to come.

"The funeral home will come. It will be a good idea for you to decide which one you will use. The funeral home will come and take the body away, and either I or Dr. Fryer will do the death certificate. And that's about that."

She exhales deeply. Not an easy conversation for any of us.

I ask, hesitantly, "Can you tell me what this will actually look like?"

"Well, there will be increased symptoms; we'll respond with increased medications; there will be decreasing sensorium, disengagement. You'll probably find that Rob will withdraw from his surroundings. He'll be less able and less interested in all those things around him. He'll take to his bed. And his body will shut down, one system at a time. He may become jaundiced; he will stop showing an interest in food and drink."

I notice the tenderness in Grace's voice. Always gentle, caring, and always truthful with the facts.

"Thanks, Grace," Rob says.

I am crying imagining all this, tears streaming down my face. I can't stop the tears and try to gather myself. I grab Kleenex after Kleenex. I am hearing over and over, "There will be increased symptoms; we'll respond with increased medications." I remember that the first forty-five minutes of this conversation was about Rob's increasing symptoms and the fact that Grace is working with the medications to try to respond. I think, *This is it. This is what is happening. She's said it will be a slow, steady decline over the course of a few weeks. We must be starting down that road, we're there.*

"So, about the CT scan next week," Grace continues. "You don't have to have one. Nobody can force you. Are you still good to go with it?"

"I think we'll still carry on," Rob says calmly.

I walk Grace to the door.

"I'll bring the paperwork next time to go through this with you. It's just paperwork, and we'll go through it and get it done," Grace says matter-of-factly.

I hear this and realize we're in a new moment, heading towards the inevitable.

Grace leaves, and I go back to the living-room where Rob is sitting.

He suggests, "Let's have a cup of tea" — English medicine for crisis and joy.

I make the tea, and we sit together quietly, in the rolling waves of the wake of this visit.

Tuesday 17 November 2009

Grace

AS I LEAVE, I take in the beautiful day outside. Driving away, I realize I am very grateful Rob asked this question. It's so difficult to make the call *when* to raise this difficult subject. Up to this point we hope for time. With less confident and capable people, broaching this topic is so difficult. Even after all these years, I still find it hard to know that right moment.

What makes some situations better or easier, and what contributes to the right timing? It was good for Jen that he asked this, but also good for me as the caregiver. It gave me permission to give the information freely, and they needed to have it. It's about mutuality of respect that Rob could raise this question. It was easier for me to talk about the practical aspects than the piece about how he'd look.

I am very glad to have had this open and honest conversation that Rob initiated. I can see it was hard for Jen, but so right, so necessary.

Wednesday 18 November 2009

Jen

I'M IN MY KITCHEN, and I call Helen to cancel our appointment on Friday. Cancelling disappoints me. I want to grab on to that experience I had last time, and now, especially, because Rob appears to be declining. We don't have much time. I desperately want to solidify this other-worldly relationship I've glimpsed with him.

"I just don't think we can see you this Friday, Helen. Rob's had a terrible week, they've booked a chest X-ray, and they think he might have clots in his lung." I'm teary telling her this.

Helen talks to me and is reassuring, kind, and a wonderful ear. I tell her, "I'm learning how to knit. I had a dream a couple of nights ago where I thought I was the one dying of cancer and that I needed to finish knitting a pair of red mittens so that Haley would have something to remember me by. At that point in the dream I realized it wasn't me that had cancer, it was Rob, and I had an overwhelming feeling of how he must feel, knowing he was going to be leaving his children. When I woke up, I asked Rob's sister-in-law Lorraine, his older brother Andrew's wife, if she would teach me how to knit. So apparently, I am knitting a scarf."

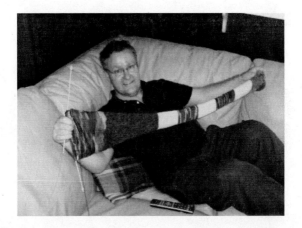

"Oh, Jen, that's wonderful!" Helen responds enthusiastically. "Knitting is such an alchemy of heart and hands. Our grandmothers poured so much of their private heartaches into knitting, quilts, and crafts. How wise those instincts are! I imagine you are feeling and carrying Rob's grief of leaving his children. You're so in tune with each other,"

She pauses. I wonder what is coming.

"I don't normally do this, Jen, but I've sat with this for a while, since our last session, and I would like to offer you the opportunity to connect via e-mail. I know you have a BlackBerry that you use often that is part of the firewalled network of our health care system, so from a privacy standpoint it seems more secure to offer you this. I know there might not be much time, and I hear you that you don't want to leave Rob's side. It's a way we can stay connected even if you can't get to my office."

What an offer! What a relief! "Thanks so much, Helen. That would be great." An e-mail connection with spiritual care! Rob's disintegrating health seems to be compromising our ability to go to appointments. The energy it takes him to go to London for chemotherapy is enormous, and he leaves the two-hour sessions exhausted.

A session with Helen in addition seems too much to ask of him. Our last session was so important. I know e-mail can't replace face to face, but it seems the next best thing. I am so thankful.

Helen

I AM GOING OUT on a limb here. I know that, from many standpoints. But again, it feels intuitively right. Jen is a professional health care provider, I know she won't abuse the offer, and it feels very important to have a way to continue this thread of support with them. They've really grabbed onto deepening their connection with one another, and it feels too soon to withdraw from my role, but there's no way they can get here to me, and phone calls are so intrusive. And I notice that Jen talks so much about the significance of the e-mails they get and how much buoyancy they receive from them. I follow my intuition, once again.

Wednesday 18 November 2009
First E-mail from Jen to Helen

> Hi Helen,
>   We had a teary night tonight. Rob had some more breakthrough
> pain today than usual and is nervous about his upcoming chest x-ray
> and C.T. scan. He's worried he's progressing, as am I, more because

time has marched on than any symptoms, but all the same, the concern is there. Tonight was the most I've seen Rob cry since the day he was diagnosed. I joked and told him it was about time.

This is my deadly time, kids and Rob in bed, I'm wandering downstairs alone, tidying up, going over the day and the tomorrows. This is when my mind turns to the future without him, it's unbearable some nights.

Our talk today was good, and I really appreciate the ability to e-mail you, thanks.

Rob was talking tonight about how he wants to write a letter to each of the four kids, and that's when he got teary saying how proud he is of all of them and how he hopes they know that. He's such a wonderful dad. I wish the little ones could have more of him, they need him so much.

Take care Helen.

Jen

Wednesday 18 November 2009
E-mail from Helen to Jen

Hi Jen,

Take care, keep writing and breathe deeply into the heartache, breathing is more medicine than we realize. Breathing with you.

Helen

P.S. I love Rob's idea of the letters and even though it may be gut wrenching for him to write them, and you to read them and go through that with him, the process itself may well be very powerful and again, the grief itself is terrifying but it is in the process of the feeling of the feelings that the healing seeds are sown and start to grow, the old cliché, the way out is the way through, being so true.

Whatever Rob's instincts guide him to do is very trustworthy.

And Jen, the knitting seems brilliant to me; a stroke of deep wisdom that is weaving something beyond your ability to know with

your mind.
    Breathing with you all ...
    Helen

Helen

WE'VE BROKEN NEW ground here is my immediate thought after sending this e-mail. We can stay in touch without its taking a toll on energy and time for them. What a gift this electronic age is.

Saturday 21 November 2009
E-mail from Jen to Grace and Helen

> *Hi Grace & Helen,*
> *I don't know who to talk to, so I thought I'd write you. I've fallen apart tonight in tears. Rob's had a rough few days with more nausea and pain than usual and I can't help but think this is the cancer eating him alive. I just tucked him in and have come downstairs, knowing I can't fall asleep right now and I can't stop the tears.*
> *I don't know how I will ever do this without him. He is my soul mate; I love him so deeply and completely. I spoke with my friend Julia on Friday night. I've known her since I was twelve, my best friend although I rarely see her in person.*
> *She told me she has meant to send a card to Rob for a while, thanking him for giving me back to her as myself. She says that when Rob and I got together, I was as she had known me when we were young.*
> *How will I ever be me again when he's gone? How will I parent effectively? How will I cope with my own grief let alone the intense grief of my kids? How will I help my step kids cope with the loss of their dad?*
> *I don't think I can. I feel so intertwined with Rob, he has always been there waiting for me to find him and when I did I completed*

so many connections I never knew existed. How will I exist without him there?

I keep thinking of never hearing his footsteps coming down the stairs, and never hearing his voice, never hearing him working on something in the basement, never whispering to him in the dark. I don't think I can do all this alone and still be me.

I'm lost, I know you can't do anything to help this but I had to connect with someone.

Jen

Saturday 21 November 2009
E-mail from Helen to Jen

Dear Jen,

I hear your heartache, Jen, and the loss of imagining 'how' in the future you will ever live through this.

I imagine I would likely feel exactly as you are describing. Lost. I am glad you can reach out and I am so very glad to be alongside you in this journey, not because I feel I have any answers in a way but because it is, in a way, teaching me too.

I hold the question with you, deeply in my heart, how can Rob's dying be a 'void' that births new life for you, for the children and for him too? Is this at all 'true' or possible? I believe in every cell of my body that it is, because the truth is 'written' throughout the body of the earth and how she lives life and death, but how it is true for you specifically and your children and Rob, that is the journey we are on together.

The truth is being written into your bodied experience with heartache, tears, gut wrenching grief, and someday, you will look back and see how Rob's death drew the deepest chasm of pain in your life and from that chasm came wisdom, love, truth, connection and life beyond your imagining in this moment.

We can never see that when we think about the future. Pain takes us into darkness only and we forget that there is never only the dark;

light is born from the void just as the baby is born from the womb of darkness into life. You could not imagine the overwhelming show of love in the cards the moment Rob was diagnosed but they came and showed him and you how deeply you are loved and respected. Life will support you in small, silent, surprising ways and it will support your children and Rob's children too.

The only way I know how to live that truth is to stay connected to your own feelings, keep grieving, keening, being real; your children will draw much from your being real in your grief. You don't have to hold it all for them; it is not all on your shoulders to figure out what they need. They will call from you what they need from you, and the rest you can let go of and trust that life will bring them and they will draw to themselves what they need.

I can offer you this Jen; you are not alone in supporting your children. Those 'beings' whoever they are that brought you and Rob together for reasons beyond your awareness are with you now, with your children and are holding you all. Life never ever abandons us, it seems that it cannot protect us from grief, sorrow, loss but it sure does show up and support us in very seemingly little ways that give us 'breadcrumbs' to take the next breath, the next step.

Keep grieving. Keep feeling.

Why Rob has to die I have no idea, Jen. I wish with all my heart it is not so. But I know with that bone deep knowing that he won't be going far at all, he will undoubtedly find ways to be present, ways you can't imagine now and that won't take away the deep, aching loss of his physical form, but you and he are on a journey of discovery about what 'life' really is and how much more than this physical form Life truly is.

You will discover his gift to you is not going to die with him. You will rise out of the ashes of grief in ways you cannot even imagine right now.

Helen

Wednesday 25 November 2009
E-mail from Jen to Grace and Helen

Hi Grace & Helen,
Its evening, Rob and kids are in bed. He had a better evening, stomach stayed settled, and no nausea since two o'clock in the afternoon.

The weight that this Christmas will hold is hitting me tonight. Rob has brought me such joy in the five Christmas seasons we've shared. He's always made it so fun for the kids. It's hard to hear everyone preparing excitedly and realize this will be such a difficult year for us. We talked a bit about it tonight and cried together. Rob so rarely cried until recently, seems to happen more freely now. He always says the same thing; that he doesn't want to leave me, it's crushing to hear.

Time is flying by so quickly. Christmas seemed so far away when he was diagnosed and was our goal to get to, it's scary to have reached it. Almost feels like the end of a rope that's been holding me up and that I've been afraid to reach.

When I first started dating Rob after the demise of my first marriage, my Mom described him as a soft spot for me to land. I feel like all the protection and comfort he's given me these years is about to be ripped from under me and my kids. I'm so desperate to hold on to him, yet I know that desperation is causing him to try and protect me by minimizing his complaints and it's only when awful symptoms like nausea show up that he lets go and bares it to me. I can't stand the thought of him not being with me through the rest of my life and my kids' lives and his kids' lives. We all need him so much.

I'm so nervous to hear the C.T. scan results, we both are. This has been such a tough week and I know they're just going to get worse.

Think that's all. Thanks for listening.
Jen

Thursday 26 November 2009
E-mail from Helen to Jen

Hi Jen,
I'm sorry Rob's struggling with the nausea, keep Grace in the loop closely, maybe she can help?
I see such raw honesty and truth in what you have the courage to name over and over about what you're living. You're being very courageous Jen, truly. It may not feel like it at all, but you are letting your grief flow, staying with your guts and the messiness of it all that takes a strength and courage even though those are the last things you probably feel right now.
Ever with you all on the heartline.
Helen

Thursday 26 November 2009
E-mail from Jen to Helen

Hi,
No, I don't feel courageous at all. Feel scared. I definitely don't feel strong; just feel like I'm going to lose it all the time.
Thanks for writing. It helps to write.
Jen

Thursday 26 November 2009
E-mail from Helen to Jen

I'm glad it helps Jen.
In my experience, my strongest times have never ever felt that at the time. So just naming the 'losing it', naming the struggle, naming the fears, 'awaring' it all with some mindful awareness; that is great strength.
You can't carry everyone's grief, children's or Rob's, for them. You

can only feel your own and let them have their feelings, staying present to each other in it. Another thing I have come to realize is that my perception of another's suffering is usually inaccurate to some degree. Not that it is 'less than' I perceive but that the same truth applies to them as it does to me or you.

Life shows up with support, with breadcrumbs, with something for them. It is true for each person that strength can be found in impossible situations and heartbreaks, somehow, unimaginably. Our minds won't ever imagine that in our 'forecasting' and perceiving of the future or another's pain, 'mind' only ever seems to imagine the horror, the fear, and the emptiness.

It is also true that none of this is meaningful in the actual experience, only retrospectively. Somehow 'wisdom' or 'truth' is not something that happens (or helps much) in the midst of the heartbreak but somehow wisdom gets forged by it. We just have to keen, grieve, wail, rage, move the pain through over and over by feeling it, banging our fists on the pillows, throwing the rocks, sobbing until you fall asleep exhausted, and somehow, through that process, wave after wave after wave, comes the experience of something beyond the pain and the abyss.

And we need to be held by others in that process. Otherwise, we can't go there deeply, it's too scary and we can feel like we're going crazy.

With energy to you on the heartline and much, much care.
Helen

Chapter 8

How Do We Do This?

∞

Jen

"GOOD NEWS, JEN, good news." Grace reads me the scan results over the telephone: "'Primary mass in pancreas has shown significant shrinkage — liver metastases are almost imperceptible.' Good call on getting the CT scan. We'll carry on!"

I feel elation.

Rob is napping. I run and wake him up and tell him the good news, hugging him. This is so thrilling. We celebrate this milestone.

A respite, a break in the speed train to his death. I'm hugging him tightly in exuberance.

"That's great. But I am still nauseous!" he says politely to my tightly hugging him.

I release him from my grip. I'm holding on to life, I'm holding on to Rob.

We celebrate with his anti-nausea pill!

Friday 27 November 2009
Third Spiritual Care Session

Helen

ONCE AGAIN I take a deep breath. Jen and Rob are coming for their third session today. Again, the feeling of empty-handed poverty. What do I possibly have to offer them? They're about to lose this incredible love they have, or its form anyway. What on earth will ameliorate such deep, anguished loss?

Again the feeling that this session might be the last: he could turn for the worse, they could decide they've gone far enough; they could cast me off as a flake. The possibilities are endless as to why we don't follow people to the end of their process, if there ever is an 'end.'

I say my usual, silent prayer, offering myself to the process, asking for inner guidance.

So, they arrive at my door on this, our third meeting.

"Hi, Jen, hi, Rob. Good to see you."

"Hello," they respond, quietly.

I notice Rob looks tired, and his face is filling out with the steroids. I don't know what he is thinking. He is so, so quiet. Jen does most of the talking. Yet she tells me how much he talks and shares with her. I know this is not the stoic person who rarely communicates anything. *Still waters run deep* is my inner sense of Rob.

He allows Jen to share their story with me — their process, how they are, conserving his energy. As she does so, I am searching with every tracking skill for fear of dying, for resistance to the inevitable of this cancer. I cannot find it, in either of them. It's quite incredible. I try hard with my well-honed nose for inner currents of lurking dread, terror, and fear that are not reaching their conscious awareness. I cannot find even a hint of them in Rob's equanimity.

Jen is definitely afraid, afraid of losing Rob in her life, but not resisting, not inwardly begging for cure and the impossible miracle. Her prayer is consistently for more time, just more time. I find this so touching and so possible. They are already presenting in a way I've never met before, so head on, so surrendering, yet without despair.

How do we do this? is their driving question. What does hope mean when one is NOT focusing on cure as the hope, whether possible or not? This is their implicit question of me as the spiritual care provider. They are not asking me to have an answer, but they are seeking guidance in how to live the question.

We move through the usual preliminaries of how they're doing, the medical story of chemotherapy leading the way. They tell me about chemotherapy and adapting to opioids for the pain, and I ask how their hearts are doing, how they are together in all this. The sharing drops to a deeper place, and they tell me they've been practising meditation with the heartline.

My ears prick up. They've been "practising"! That means they're taking what I said very seriously. Suddenly, I am aware again of what a terrible set-up this will be if I am wrong. What if I've led them down the garden path of false hope, a band-aid, out of my own desire to 'help' them in their suffering? But, once again, my bones tell me to keep going.

"So what have you been experiencing?" I ask.

"Well, I feel him, I definitely feel him. And he is a sort of yellow energy in my mind's eye," says Jen.

"You too, Rob?" I ask, looking at him very directly.

Rob nods in agreement.

I notice my desire to hear more of Rob's voice in the room, to understand what is going on in his depths, what he is feeling and experiencing. And also, to understand how on earth a man of forty-six, with a family, can be facing his death with such incredible and seemingly authentic equanimity when he hasn't been a practising Buddhist, nor a native elder, nor a Christian contemplative.

Rob is a mystery to me, and I really want to understand how he is doing this. I have met no one, in five years of cancer care or ten years in health care, with this quality of spirit in the face of their mortality at such a young age. I have seen it in the last days of a person's life, when often a peacefulness settles in, but he is possibly months away from dying. How is he living this?

"Yes, I feel Jen very much." His Scouse accent, lacing his words, stirs great affection for my own English roots. His response is, as usual, succinct, to the point, and leaves me wishing he'd say more.

He's like a living Buddha flies across my mind. Rob, in his 'is-ness,' is like a peaceful Buddha.

"Would you like to share another meditation then and keep exploring this?" I ask.

I have absolutely no idea whatsoever what I am going to offer them.

They nod vigorously. "Yes, we would very much. It was very powerful last time."

I invite them to put their feet on the ground. I plant my own firmly, for I need to find my centre to dive into this.

We feel the earth beneath our feet. I guide us into simple awareness of breath, of feet on the earth, of the deep soil of the earth beneath the layers of concrete, of the trees surrounding us in the earth sharing our breath. The first peoples of Turtle Island, which is what its native peoples call North America, offer us the wisdom and teachings that cultivate a sense of deep interconnection with life's web. In fact, they teach us that we forget this at our peril.

Simply breathing with the trees is a profound practice for many people, along with the feeling of their own feet on the earth, imagining roots boring down into the soil. This ancient Celtic meditation would take place in the oak groves of Cornwall, Ireland, Scotland, and Wales and is a very potent way to reconnect with the deep and ancient river of wisdom coursing through our veins in our own blood and bones.

Now, I invite them to imagine a place in nature again, which I introduced in our second session, to go there in their mind's eye, feel it with all their senses, take in the medicine of that sacred place that has called them in nature.

I ask them where they are. They are both at the beach. A beach they love and have been to. Out of the blue comes the portal into what this meditation is about, where it is taking us. I see it and dive in before I have time to second guess myself.

"So, imagine the rocks that this beach used to be. Think of the time every grain of sand has lived through and the changes that they have undergone. Think of how, millennia ago, this sand was rocks, cliffs, that were weathered by the ice, rain, wind, waves and slowly over thousands, millions of years were worked upon by the elements of the forces of life to become the sand you are now walking on.

"And see in your mind's eye where those cliffs came from — the very centre, the bowels of the earth — that they were once molten, red hot lava, liquid, moving in the earth's core until she erupted and spewed her essence out into the air to become the mountains and cliffs that were worn down over time to become the sand.

"And before they were lava, what were they? Where do the rocks begin? Can we ever actually pinpoint where something begins?

"If we go back in time before the earth was the earth as we know it, what was she before this form? Meteors? Energy fields spewing from perhaps the big bang that created all this that we are?

"Where does life begin? Where does it end? Forms end, forms change, life is ever changing, but always essence is the same, the same life force morphing, growing, dying, evolving into the next form. The rocks are alive, they are being rocks, and the sand is 'sanding,' or being sand.

"As you walk on this beach of sand, as you are in these forms of your bodies, as they are right now, think of where you came from. Think of how you met, how your paths led you to that first meeting. What were the chances of that happening? You could have been sick on the day of the workshop. You may never have crossed paths, but you did.

"And then the time it took through dissolving marriages to stumble upon the deep love that drew you eventually into being each other's beloved. Your paths weaving, ever weaving into the deep love you now share, your lives comingled and entwined into 'this' that you feel in your bones even now, with death on your shoulder.

"And what is death? Did the lava die when it spewed into the air and hardened into mountains? Did they die when they became rocks broken down by ice and rain? Did they die when they dissolved into sand, beaten by waves over and over? Are the waves beating the shore or making love to it? How can we know?

"Our minds simply label what we've been conditioned to believe. Is the gazelle killed by the tiger, or is it giving its life to feed the life-cycle by offering itself, as indigenous people often teach? They've studied life in front of their eyes; their schools were the school of life around them, instead of reading about it in books. We've lost touch with that wisdom.

"What is death? Do we ever really die, or do we simply change forms and become something else? Where do we end? Where does life begin?"

I can feel the pulsing inwardly of a guided process. It's a feeling of being in a river, and I am simply following the current, carried, allowing it to move me. No two meditations are every exactly the same. I respond to an inner momentum, images emerging in my mind's eye, creating a narrative. I can name it only as energy, a force that is I but not I, a feeling I have learned to trust.

In the silence, I can feel Rob and Jen's concentration, the shared synergy of this moment, our interconnection. They are right with me in this meditation; I do not have to open my eyes to know that.

I pause, wondering, *What now? Where do we go now?*

Then the portal opens, and the way forward becomes clear. Shape shifting. A term I experienced through Arnold Mindell, another weaving on my path in recent years, now feeding into this moment. I am about to offer something I've never suggested before.

"Rob, I want you to imagine that you are a shape shifter, because we all are. Shamans would and can shape shift into different forms to go on their spirit journeys for healing and for wisdom for the tribe. A shaman would become an eagle and take flight and go on a spirit journey. Let something in this beach call you, and practise shape shifting into that form. Become whatever it is that calls you, feel yourself changing shape, and feel it in your fingers, in your toes.

"Relate with Jen through that form with your essence. Imagine what it's like to feel her as 'that' thing — that you've become that life form and part of the earth. Notice that this is exactly what has happened; you've simply morphed into another energetic form that is in fact, in essence, the same energy you are in your body as 'Rob.'

"And so, in your death, this is simply what will happen; a becoming of another form with which you will learn to relate with Jen. Feel her; reach out to her with all that love in your heart and body, but as that other form you've become."

I pause, to let him take his own time in this rather startling idea, which I certainly have never tried before. I wonder whether Rob is in any way able to experience what I've suggested. I feel into the energy in the room. It's palpably deep and rich and connected. I know he's with me in this, but how, and what he's experiencing, I've no idea.

"Now, slowly, bring yourself back into the form that is this body for now. This 'Rob' that you are in this moment in time. Bring yourselves back to awareness of your body in this room, feel the couch under you, another form of energy that right now is 'couch' but before was chemicals, liquid soup, and wood that was trees. Be aware of each other's presence in the room, and, when you're ready, open your eyes and come back to this moment in time."

Slowly, they open their eyes. The old, familiar reorienting to the now that happens after a deep and present meditation. They look at each other and smile a brief smile.

A silence that feels very hallowed hangs in the air.

"What did you notice happening?" I ask them. My curiosity piqued with slight anxiety, because I'd just dived right off the deep end. They are after all, along with being patients, health care professionals in my own hospital network. This could have reverberations beyond these four walls.

"It was very good," says Rob, simply. Jen nods her agreement.

This time I don't let him off the hook with his succinctness.

"What did you notice happen that felt good for you?" I ask ... yes, prodding. I am very aware that I am prodding. I need to know. I can't know where to go if I don't know what happened in the current moment and where this has taken them both.

"Well, I liked the meditation with the rocks and cliffs and sand," Rob begins. "I've never thought about time in that way before, and it's true, you can't pinpoint when it all begins. Just always changing."

I did not know then that Rob was an avid hiker in England, with a great love of the craggy hills and rocks of our homeland, as was I. My instinct to go to the rocks was accurate, an image that is alive for him.

"And what happened when I suggested you shape shift into another form? What did you notice then?" I am being very careful indeed to keep it as open-ended as possible.

"I became the sand," he responds, with a moving simplicity and real-ness. "I could feel her on me as the sand; I was supporting Jen, from underneath her." Rob gestures while cupping his hands, as if cupping something above them.

I feel the tears pricking my eyes. What a gift to Jen. She'll never experience sand in the same way again after he's died. If nothing else, if he never 'exists' after death, and all this is just wishful thinking, she'll always have sand — she'll always have him with her, experientially, under her feet, under her body, whenever she walks or lies on sand. The beach can be a refuge for her. I am so grateful.

Jen looks at him. "I could feel you very strongly. I could feel you with me, around me."

"Do you have any image in mind when you're feeling Rob?" I ask. I've heard Jen talk enough to know that she loves images and often speaks with metaphor quite naturally.

"He's yellow, like light, a yellow energy. Quite bright," she responds.

What a relief! The deep end we've dived into has held us all up! Something has happened here that is as profound as it is real. I am perhaps not off my rocker, and the risks, professional and personal, have been worth it. I am following something whose name no longer matters, but a reality that is as alive and real as my hand in front of me and is giving this young couple, facing death in their lives, a possibility of a connection that will transcend Rob's physical dying. I am overwhelmed and grateful for what has happened in this room today.

They are too.

"So, Rob, this is your practice. This is your time of strengthening what the Buddhists would call your 'energy body' for the dying of the mortal body. They have a five-thousand-year-old wisdom passed from master to student by 'transmission,' which is what you've just experienced. A transmission from life itself, from whatever guides are guiding us, to teach you about this reality, this inner, invisible reality. You are training to become a shape shifter par excellence, so that, when you die, you simply morph into another form and retain your essence and this deep love of the two of you remains strong and interconnected.

"I believe it's possible. You've just tasted what that's like. Now it's about practising and learning to open your minds and hearts to this other reality that has been guarded and held in awareness by peoples in different cultures across the planet.

"And Jen," I continue, "you can practise feeling Rob, tuning in, as it were, to his essence from a distance. When you're falling asleep, perhaps together, practise knowing how to feel his energetic identity and essence."

I can see the sadness still coursing through Jen's face. Yes, that's the thing with these inner experiences. They do not gloss over the pain of the loss. If they do, they're not the real deal. Pain is the portal, there is no way out, only through — it's the eye of the needle. The reality of the inner world and its depth of wisdom will support us, if we can but listen, trust it.

Rob seems very content with the experience. The same equanimity, the same quiet and absolute presence.

It felt important. It felt right. What will happen from this, I have no idea.

The session has reached its natural endpoint, and right on time. We say our goodbyes as they leave this 'other world' within the world of the cancer program and head out of my room.

Trusting one's bones can take one into some strange places.

Jen

IN THE DAYS AND WEEKS that follow, Rob and I take this practice as our essential work. I practise feeling his energy, feeling into him when he is sleeping as I am busy around the house. I crawl into bed next to him, wrap my arm around him, and practise feeling his energy.

Some nights, if he is awake, I ask him, "Can we do that thing that Helen did?"

He replies, quite simply, "I am."

And if he is asleep, I do it anyway. It becomes our nightly ritual for the rest of our time together and beyond.

The first meeting with Helen and the next two meditation sessions developing the heartline with her kick-start a process that we grab onto and run with. We are counting days; I am desperately hoping to reach Christmas, begging for time from the universe. Our children need time.

The practice evolves gradually. I see if I can tune into Rob's cancer and send messages to the cancer, keep it at bay, and let the chemotherapy find the cancer cells. Or, Where are you, Rob? Is your essence in there, in the midst of all this cancer?

I always find him, feel him. I ask for more time, always, amid a flood of welling tears. I let the tears come, and I then feel as if hands are taking my shoulders, and I hear the words, OK. You've got time.

The peaceful feeling I had while on my knees crying in the living-room, five days after his diagnosis, happens over and over when I practise connecting with Rob's energy — my attempt to meditate and connect with this invisible realm. Often I lie next to him at night sobbing.

"Just stay," I beg.

"I am. I'm not going anywhere." He holds me, and the same peaceful feeling comes over me. His words fill me with calm. Always Rob is calm.

Saturday 28 November 2009
Rob Update

We've had quite a roller coaster of a few weeks since I wrote last. What was supposed to be our week off chemotherapy ended up being full of medical appointments. Rob had been experiencing some chest tightness and a few other symptoms (nausea, ankle swelling, sort of like being pregnant) that caused our palliative care doc to query pulmonary embolism week before last. Blood clots are a common complication of pancreatic cancer apparently.

All the tests thankfully came back clear, no clots in legs or lungs. We then had our monthly oncologist appointment this past Monday and then a C.T. scan Tuesday. The C.T. scan was the first one since he was diagnosed, and was ordered by the oncologist to "see what the cancer is doing". What a terrifying test that was to prepare for. Neither of us slept very well the night before.

It was not a fun day. We were forewarned at our appointment with the oncologist on Monday to not worry about the C.T. scan, that we should brace ourselves for the cancer to have grown. The oncologist has always said that the chemotherapy was to produce subjective improvement, so less pain, less nausea, more energy (all of which it has done) and that the gemcitabine rarely produces objective improvement, meaning that it would not cure the cancer, just make Rob feel a bit better. Rob is the barometer that will determine whether we continue with chemotherapy, it has to make sense for him.

We got the results of the C.T. scan back on Thursday and surprise, surprise, the tumours have actually shrunk! Many of them have shrunk as much as two thirds, the main one in the pancreas by one third. Obviously we were very pleased, as was our super duper nurse practitioner and the oncologist.

As exciting as this is, it's quickly tempered by the message that the cancer will eventually grow even with chemotherapy, it will develop a 'resistance' to gemcitabine but, for now, this is nice news and we see this as an indication that we will have some more months together.

The oncologist actually seemed somewhat surprised at the tumour shrinkage. I don't know if it's the floods of positive energies that people send our way through cards and e-mails, the prayers said at various church congregations, or bedsides, or desks, or physio gyms (I know I pray in the strangest places these days, often in the ladies room at the cancer clinic!), the Essiac tea that I cook like a witch every few weeks, or just Rob's incredible will and perseverance to stay present with his family, but something in addition to chemotherapy has got to be at play here. I believe it in my bones.

As nice as all the diagnostic test results have been these last few days, Rob has unfortunately felt quite ill, he's been quite nauseous for the past week and a half. We're mid way through trying some different combinations of anti-emetic drugs to combat the nausea and luckily Dr. Fryer is not satisfied to have him live with the nausea, she's determined she can somehow get rid of it. Rob's now taking thirty-one pills a day, more on the days around chemotherapy.

Tomorrow we're trying acupuncture from a physiotherapist friend of ours to see if that helps the nausea, we may move to 'pot in a pill', the pharmaceutical marijuana derivatives. I can't imagine Rob mellower than he already is, might be an interesting Christmas! The nice thing is it's easier to put up with the nausea if you know the chemotherapy that is likely causing it is also doing some good.

Sunday 29 November 2009
E-mail from Helen to Jen

Hi Jen,
Thank goodness for Grace. I must say, you've drawn around you
so many resources, that is a mirror of who you are in life and how
some part of you, even in the midst of devastation such as when the
diagnosis first happened, mobilizes and draws support and resourc-
es towards yourselves. Take heart from that. It's happening despite
the feeling that there is so little strength within for this journey.
A practice that I want to share more with you both is called the
practice of awareness or as one teacher calls it 'awaring' because it's
not a state of being but an active practice that is deceivingly simple
but the only antidote I know to tackle that mind of ours which just
runs off like a wild horse out of the gate charging into the horror
stories of the future and the only antidote and practice that helps to
deal with powerful emotions.
Simply put, and we've done a bit of it in our sessions, it's the
practice of putting your mind to work on the present moment rather
than the future. It will live in the future given half the chance, and
this kind of experience, the anticipation of a traumatic loss, already
begun in a way, is probably the most difficult experience to rein in in
your mind and make it work FOR you instead of against you.
And planning for the future is very different from the creation of
terrifying stories about the future.
Ever with respect and trust in what we call 'life' to support and
guide you both.
Helen

Tuesday 1 December 2009
E-mail from Jen to Helen

Hi Helen,
I'm going to try and go to bed soon but wanted to write to you.
Another round of chemotherapy has started, Rob's nausea has settled

a little with a new med regime from Grace, thank goodness for her.

I'm finding the positive C.T. results have left me a little unsettled feeling, possibly that there is a backtracking, or rest in the roll down the hill of impending doom? Not sure. I read the survivor stories on pan can (a pancreatic cancer website) for the first time in a couple of months, found a story similar to ours with a happy ending. Then abruptly switched off the computer; almost felt mad at myself for thinking such a thing and 'jinxing' it, which makes me feel like I'm twelve.

As I said, unsettled, because an hour earlier I was sobbing as I left the bedroom having tucked Rob into bed, and telling him he just had to stay because so many people needed him; which makes me feel guilty, because if he had anything to do with it he wouldn't leave; which is maybe why he hasn't so far. He probably has a lot more to do with the outcome than my science brain would let me believe.

I read your long e-mail out loud to Rob this afternoon, you sent it before I picked up the kids from school.

One thing I would really like more help on: the first time Rob and I came in together you led us through a meditation where we tried to 'feel' each other's energy and focus on images. I felt Rob that day, I know I did, and I'd like to learn from you while he's still here and can come with me to your office how to do that.

I can't remember when you work on Wednesdays, but I'll try and get in touch with you at work and see if we can squeeze something in before Christmas. I'd like to. Needing sleep. I'll talk to you soon. I'm knitting a scarf. It's two thirds done. Maybe Rob will wear it to your office one day.

Take care. Thank you for what you're doing.

Jen

Wednesday 2 December 2009
E-mail from Helen to Jen

Hi Jen,

There is something so wonderful about the scarf. I can't put my finger on it but it is somehow its own alchemy and medicine.

I notice you've named a few times feeling guilty for speaking your truth to Rob about not wanting him to leave. I personally have this gut response that says it's a good thing that you do. The energy of withholding that feeling in the speaking of it would be so draining and felt in the air anyway. Allowing 'what is' to be alive lets the energy of it take us and move us somewhere else, even if it repeats over and over. In the end, we'll end up somewhere else; but not if we stifle our truth and feelings.

I am happy to keep working together on practicing connecting energetically.

Yes, awaring. If it takes years in the ancient monastic traditions for buddhist monks to learn it, without raising children and having meals cooked for them I think we can have some grace for ourselves for finding it strange, difficult and like working a muscle we've never used, because it is. I do find a little often goes a long way and while it doesn't change the emotions or stop them, it does change the experience of them even if it is just by a hair and that can make all the difference.

It's also very self-nurturing and supportive of your body and heart because you're giving attentiveness to your own heart/body/mind by practicing it with the breath and turning your attention to your experience instead of getting so utterly lost within the wave of emotion. That happens but over time, there is 'catching' oneself that comes quicker and easier, not to snuff or prevent the tidal wave of emotion but to hold ourselves very gently in it.

This respite in the progress of Rob's tumours is a trustworthy gift of some nature. Whatever is in the future, this moment, right now, there is breath, presence, relationship and as hard as it is to drag your mind off and away from the future keep dragging it back to the here and now where he is, with you. And this is so easy to say and so ultimately almost impossible to do, but the trying is the important thing. He is still here with you, trust that these moments you have now, are for a reason that will serve you in some way when the time comes that he is not, whenever that is.

Each moment now, metabolizing and changing something about what that time will be like for you, whether that's because you are strengthening your energetic connection with him now, or whether you're gaining some inner strength without realizing it, whether Rob's working on things inwardly that may never be visible, even to himself. Who knows, but each moment has a purpose to it and has all of time wrapped up in it, past, present, and future.

This love you've co-created together is timeless, belongs in a realm that isn't measured by time and space; a field of energy that exists beyond your individual 'sum of your parts.' Your children are in that field, part of it. That love exists whether your bodies are breathing or not.

You can't see right now, how that is very, very Real. Your love, dare I put a capital on it; that Love will seep and permeate the whole journey you are on, each of you in your family, and some of what that means cannot be seen while the physical body is still alive. Some of what Love creates and permeates into our bones, adult and child, can't be seen until a loved one becomes invisible.

I wouldn't wish having to grapple with whether this is true, or real on anyone. I so wish it wasn't happening to you and Rob, with all my heart. Yet, I truly trust the realness of the love you share. It's big and will be there for you Jen, even in the midst of all the sobs and heartbreak. You won't lose his love or the Love that you've co-created and been guided by to be together.

Wrapping you all in my heart closely.
Helen

Wednesday 9 December 2009
E-mail from Helen to Jen

Hi Jen,
In true 'synchronistic' fashion I am reading our school's biannual magazine and suddenly see this paragraph which I can't even find the beginning of the article, as this part is a carryover from another

page (which eludes me). But Rudolf Steiner was the founder of Waldorf education and was a big influence in a nineteenth century intellectual and spiritual movement called 'anthroposophy' integrating humanism, philosophy, theology and anthropology (I think) anyway, he was very much a 'giant' thinker of his time and influenced medicine, farming, education, to name a few fields he got into. I offer it to ponder together in this journey we are all on.

The quote is thus… "Rudolf Steiner spoke of the dead as the 'so called dead.' He asserted that those who have passed over continue to be active in the work and affairs of the world, particularly when the living cultivate a relationship with them. In the ninety years of Waldorf education, countless dedicated Waldorf teachers have crossed the threshold from the material to the spiritual world. They have gone before us, but now follow, accompany and help us every day. Maintaining our connection to those who have crossed the threshold is crucial to our success, in our daily teaching and in the broader work for the renewal of education."

While in health care we don't run across this kind of perspective much, I am discovering more and more there is a wealth of people 'out there' who live, practice and believe this wholeheartedly and have story after story to substantiate their beliefs. I am joining them slowly as I walk with more people closely in the crossing over. Curious timing to read this today given that I don't always get to read this publication.

Take care and looking forward to reconnecting in person on Friday.

Helen

Wednesday 9 December 2009
E-mail from Jen to Grace

Hi Grace,
Certainly don't risk life and limb for us, tomorrow, if the weather is iffy, we can do the visit by phone.

Helen sent me a quote tonight about the 'so called dead' by the founder of the Waldorf education system, Rudolf Steiner. It was about the connection that can be made with those people who have died, or 'passed over'. What an interesting quote. I have this funny series of thoughts whenever I ponder what Helen or others have said about the concept of connection with those who have 'passed over', or 'heart-lines'. My initial gut reaction is that of interest and comfort, thinking that perhaps I can still have a connection with Rob, who I care for so fiercely and deeply in my bones, once his body has died. It's what I wish for; for the void not to come, for him not to entirely leave and somehow still be here with me.

Then I think of the other people in my life who have died. Both of my grandmothers for instance and I think of how I don't feel much of a connection to them at all and do feel simply that they're gone and then I well up thinking that I will someday feel that Rob is just gone and I can't face the thought of it.

Take care, Grace.

Jen

CHAPTER 9

We Make It to Christmas!

Wednesday 9 December 2009
E-mail from Jen to Helen and Grace

Hi guys,
We put up our Christmas tree tonight; a rare occurrence of all four
children home, and together putting up ornaments. An eclectic mix of
ornaments, made by them, or collected, or passed on from grandpar-
ents. A very mismatched beautiful tree.
Rob and I participated a bit then sat back and watched the family
we have created work together on probably Rob's last Christmas tree.
We had Christmas music, British hits, and auld langs aye (have no idea
how to spell that) with the lord's prayer in place of the traditional words.
Rob got very teary and upset in front of the kids. He almost panicked
with the emotion, it was heart breaking. The little ones looked worried. I
let the moment hang a bit, and then rescued him with some humour that
broke the moment. Something about the Methodist Church upbringing
and the Lord's Prayer; it was a tough night for both of us.
He was teary several more times after that, saying this may be the
last tree he puts up. Christmas is just a day, but the whole season will be
so difficult in so many ways. The mind sabotages us so often.
Take care,
Jen

Thursday 10 December 2009
E-mail from Helen to Jen

Hi Jen,

How utterly bitter-sweet the Christmas season must be for you. Bravo on your instincts of letting the grief spill and then shifting the energy for the family. You're wise woman self rising up in the moment, knowing what to do; remember how you couldn't imagine how you'd handle such a moment a month ago? You did, beautifully. That's the part of you that you can trust. You can just trust she's there when you need her and if you feel lost, overwhelmed, stay with that experience until she finds her way, because she will.

I see the wise woman in you showing up to support you so much; the dream, the knitting, the finding of all the supports that you have, the wisdom in the tree decorating moment. You are not quite so lost as you feel you are but you can't see that directly and never will, you can't see your own strength and wisdom directly and never will, but over time, you may come to trust that it's there and will support you in ways you need when you need it.

Take care and thank you, as I said, this is a journey we are all on together, a privilege and a purpose of its own in ways we don't know but are there.

Helen

Sunday 13 December 2009
E-mail from Jen to Helen

Hi Helen,

I'm sending a picture of Rob wearing my latest knitting creation; it's a bobble hat for Haley. She made the pompom. I just finished the hat tonight. I think Rob looks smashing in it.

We keep talking about the session a couple weeks ago about the sand. Rob has talked about it a lot, more so than other sessions. He says my energy body is white and his is yellow (his was yellow in my mind as well, although I was grey). He also tells me that he imagines himself as sand forming around me as he goes to sleep at night. I think this is so neat that he is willing to take these ideas and images we 'metabolize' in your office and bring them home. Never thought either of us could do that.

We've finished painting the living room and dining room and have re-assembled the room; looks beautiful. We painted it appropriately, a sand colour. It's just so important to do home renovations during a terminal illness!! It keeps us doing something together anyway.

I have discovered in painting and knitting that I need a physical project to pour energy into, it helps a lot. I hope it's not just distracting me away from reality. I don't want to hide from what's right in front of me. I don't think so though. I think doing something physical, particularly when it's a house project that we've always talked about doing (house projects have been our collective hobby for many years) gives me something to do with my hands while my head sorts through things.

I had a dream about a week ago that has stuck with me. In the dream I was exploring a new drug that may be used for cancer and trying to figure out how to get the doctor to get it for Rob, as it was experimental. I woke up with a start with the Beatles song "Let It Be" in my head and it's been there ever since. Although I'm married to a Liverpool boy, I'm not a big fan of the Beatles, and don't listen to their music regularly, but I think my mind playing the song for me was a message and I find it relaxing and sad at the same time when I stop and listen. I'd love to know what you think of all that.

I'm casting on one hundred new stitches for Jack's hat; my next project.

Thanks always for everything Helen.

Did I ever tell you my grandma, the knitter, was Helen? Helen Margaret Haley (Haley was my mom's maiden name and my daughter's name). She went by Rita. She was a war bride from Northern Ireland. Used a lot of phrases that Rob (and possibly you) use. Interesting.

Take care,

Jen

Saturday 19 December 2010
Reflections

Helen

WHAT I DID NOT KNOW during that first visit with Jen and Rob, and I know now, is that Rob in fact had a very deep belief in the energy of life that was interconnected. As a physiotherapist, he had developed his own unique method of assessment and treatment. Although he based it on conventional therapies, he had an innate skill at knowing people's potential and drawing it out. He had achieved startling and remarkable results to which observers had more than once attached the word 'miracle.'

Rob, unbeknownst to me, understood this world of connection, and I was unwittingly speaking his language, right into the heart of his belief system. It was just not a belief system he'd applied specifically to the realm of death, with the notion of sustaining relationship and interconnection beyond the grave. Yet the groundwork for him to grab onto this wholeheartedly was there.

The ecosystem that Jen, Rob, and I formed in that first meeting meant that Rob's beliefs evoked my own, without his saying a word. Their need for 'hope' — authentic, genuine hope — evoked my deepest authenticity, which meant I shared my deepest self with them, the self that holds those beliefs and intuitions close to my chest, and drew them out, despite all my professional judgments and normal resistance to sharing my personal beliefs with people, especially in an initial visit.

Yet the alchemy between us constellated the depths that wanted to speak to them, and the depths spoke and offered up a jewel that gave them something to take away, something that made them — for the first time since the devastating day of diagnosis — turn their hearts *towards* life and the time they still had together.

They had embraced death fully. Almost too fully. I had rarely met two people — a couple — who both so wholeheartedly accepted the fatality of the news with realism and utter non-resistance. Neither did I detect fatalism. They had not lain down waiting for him to die either. They just could not see any way to live with any hope, because they had no idea what to hope for.

The drawing out of the idea of the heartline and the possibility that this relationship might be able to transcend the grave became the sliver of hope they were looking for, and it gave them a project to work on together during the days, hours, and minutes of treatment that could buy only time, not cure.

Rob was very quietly, very persistently, pulling Jen along that path of his own of many years deep in his being, almost unconscious even to him until the cancer hit him. He had grabbed on to this notion I had offered with the language and concept of the heartline, and he wasn't letting it go because he wasn't letting Jen go. His love for her was so deep, so solid, that he knew this was their best shot — an arrow that was going to have to arc over death and into the great beyond, about which no one on this side can reliably talk with any authenticity. He was staking everything on it and quietly practising his own inner meditation to open his inner eyes, heart, and mind to an invisible reality that would connect Jen with him and him with her.

Wednesday 30 December 2009
Rob Update

Rob is part way through his fifth cycle of chemotherapy. He had chemotherapy last Wednesday (December twenty third) and again today, with one more next Wednesday and then we're done another cycle. Since last update he has been feeling much better. After three weeks of nausea and occasional vomiting, the doctors and nurse practitioner made some medication tweaks that worked, and have meant that chemotherapy is much smoother. The chemotherapy is doing what it needs to do for now. We are very blessed.

We have had a very busy and meaningful Christmas. We hosted a Christmas party for a few close friends the weekend before Christmas. It was wonderful. Our home was filled with Christmas carols played on our piano by a very talented friend, and we got to enjoy a few hours of festivity, where we felt like our old selves.

Rob was so energized by the event. We worried prior to the get togeth-

· er that he wouldn't be well enough to host, but he was, and it was so great to see. The amount of support and kindness and love that filled our home for those few hours was tangible. We are so grateful to have had the party.

Our Christmas was busy. We planned ahead of time to host our extended family Christmas here at our home to avoid travelling, which is never the best right after chemotherapy. Rob's parents flew in from England for their third visit since August on December twenty second, so we had Rob's parents, my parents, my brother and his family (three kids age six and under) and our four kids. It was chaotic and busy, but nice to have everyone together.

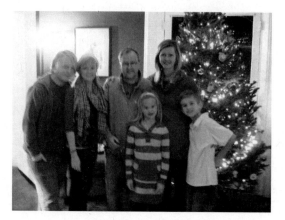

The approach to Christmas, trimming the tree, etc. was difficult for Rob and I (and all of us I expect) as there is a heaviness in the air knowing this may well be Rob's last Christmas. So in some ways the chaos in our house on Christmas day took the focus off the obvious.

We have experienced so much generosity this Christmas. Christmas baking has arrived at our door from neighbours, we have received so many beautifully written Christmas cards, and many people have donated financially to our family to help. This never ceases to amaze us when it happens. The generosity and kindness of others has been overwhelming.

A few of our close friends collected the one hundred and fifty or so cards that we have been receiving since August and have scrapbooked them. Not being a 'scrap-booker', I had no idea what this may look like, just knew I needed to uncover my dining room table prior to Christmas. We now have three beautiful leather bound large scrap books full of the most precious words and memories. They are an art form.

I never thought they would be as beautiful as they are and they brought tears to my eyes as soon as I opened the first one up. I know they will be some of my most treasured possessions for the rest of my life. They are filled with words of support and love and encouragement from the people who care about Rob and me the most, our family and friends. What a gift. Thank you.

As we approach the New Year it feels strange. New Year's for us has always meant setting a plan for the upcoming year, which this year is an impossibility. We are so grateful for Rob's well being at the moment, but can't ever count on that for any period of time, as all the medical people keep reminding us.

We have had to learn to adjust our goals to 'short term' plans, which are a challenge for both of us. Before our Christmas party, our short term goal was to paint the living and dining room (why not?). We did, it looks great. We're now moving to repainting a pantry and hall, then kitchen, and also planning a short getaway to Great Wolf Lodge with the little kids and my parents in late January. That's as far as we dare plan. Rob's short term goal is to see a golf course this spring. I bought him a new six iron in early December. He promised me he'd try it out in the spring and he's never broken a promise yet!

At the beginning of this journey, when we first heard the diagnosis, I prayed Rob would see Christmas and I thought it was a long shot from what we were told. He is full of surprises. Christmas gets many of us nostalgic for miracles and a bit spiritual, and I can't help but believe that the prayers and words of support that are contained in the words in our scrapbooks and people's homes and churches have made a difference. Please keep them coming, they are more powerful than anyone can believe.

Many thanks for everything.

Happy New Year to everyone.

Jen

Part Three

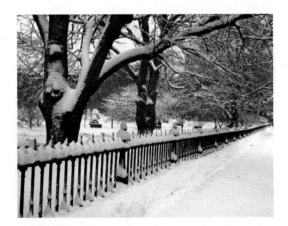

Winter 2010

CHAPTER 10

From Sprint to Marathon

∞

Early January 2010

Jen

MY MORNING ROUTINE is always the same. It's an art form I developed and perfected in the first few weeks after Rob's diagnosis in August.

I wake him up today as I do every morning at seven. I bring him a tray in bed — his first deluge of pills and a small amount of breakfast with a cup of tea. Then, our morning check-in. Our conversation this morning is good.

"How are you doing, sweetheart?" I ask, as I help him sit up on the side of the bed.

"Not bad at all. Good today," Rob, as always, in the present. No mention of yesterday ... or of tomorrow.

"How's your pain? Any nausea?"

"No pain. No nausea. Good today."

Thank God for all the drugs. This chemical soup has been a tough recipe to perfect, so much trial and error. Rob looks weary, but smiles as he eats his breakfast, and swallows thirteen pills. It will be a good day, I think.

Rob finishes his breakfast, and I tuck him back into bed for a couple more hours of much-needed rest with a hug and a kiss. I swallow hard as I leave the room. How many more times will I get to kiss him? Tears well up for the gazillionth time, the emotion washes over me, and then passes.

I've been learning to 'ride these waves' and discovering they do indeed pass, if I let them come through me. I go and get Jack and Haley up for school, always with the goal of keeping the morning routine with them *quiet,* so Rob can sleep.

I call my Mom at five after nine, right after I've dropped the kids off at school. Today has been smooth so far, and Rob is still sound asleep.

"Hello?"

"Hi, Mom."

"Hi, Jen, how's Rob today?" she asks in a fast, low whisper. Mom and I have also developed a routine. She e-mails me at about seven-thirty each morning, always the same brief message on my BlackBerry, "Hi, Jen, how's Rob today?" First contact of the day is always by e-mail. She never presumes to phone in the morning in case things are not going well. I respond every day by phone.

"He seems good today. Says he has no pain and no nausea. He's had a couple good days in a row now." I reply. I am nervous of ever admitting out loud that things are going "well," knowing this can turn within minutes, but today I offer this.

"I think he's had a good few weeks, hasn't he?" she asks.

"Yes, I guess he has. Things seem different now since Christmas. We actually reached the goal of Christmas. It feels like we're living with a whole new horizon in front of us. Rob says we're in 'bonus time' now," I remark, remembering his comment the previous evening.

"I think you are. He's doing well, Jen. And he may continue to do well for a while still," she pauses. I am quiet. She continues, "Maybe you need to look at this as 'chronic,' instead of acute. I know pancreatic cancer is an acute illness, but maybe you need to shift your thinking about how you manage it, and yourselves. He's already gone on for five months and … "

I interrupt, reacting to hope for long-term, 'chronic' timelines.

"The statistics are pretty cut and dry, Mom. This won't go on forever. This can change so quickly. We have been told that so many times. Rob and I both know that. This is not about timelines anymore. 'Bonus time' is one day at a time. I think it's a matter of shifting how we look at things.

"We spent the past five months waiting to get to Christmas. Now we've passed it. We have to change our focus, take it away from the destination and focus on the journey. I think we need to shift from running a sprint to running a marathon and accept that we just don't know how long the marathon is." I pause, realizing, "I just don't know how exactly to do that."

"You and Rob will figure it out, Jen," my Mom responds, trying to encourage me. "You've already started."

January 2009
A Port-a-cath?

THERE WERE A DIMINISHING number of nurses who could tap into Rob's veins for chemotherapy. During the Christmas holidays one of them asked, "Have you ever thought about getting a PICC line?" — a peripherally inserted central catheter. Tapping into Rob's veins was taking more heat packs, more time, more poking. The main veins in his arms were shot, and I could see that this was going to become a big problem sooner rather than later; and sooner still seemed like it existed. Rob was moving past the prognostic expectations. It was already early January.

I ask Grace next visit, "What can you tell me about central lines?"

We are sitting, as always with her, on the big couch in our living-room. Rob is in his favourite spot, where he can stretch out his legs on the sectional.

Grace replies, "I'll get back to you on the specifics, but … " She goes on to explain the options, "a PICC or a more permanent port-a-cath, while knowing that operative risks make the latter unlikely for a person with metastatic pancreatic cancer. Rob clearly needs something for his veins."

Grace explains, "Port-a-caths involve surgery, general anaesthesia, and you need a referral to the surgeon."

"It's getting more and more difficult to find veins," I respond.

Grace goes over the risks of the anaesthesia and the process. "We often put port-a-caths in kids when we know that they have several cycles of chemotherapy ahead of them."

Grace is also aware of an ethical issue about scarce resources: the devices are costly, requiring a surgeon, surgery time, general anaesthetic, and therefore an anaesthetist. In systemic decision-making, people with only weeks or months to live don't usually qualify.

"Well, I think we're facing down something here. We're going to have to do something," I push, sensing that we have another challenge ahead. "Grace, please tell me, what would you do, PICC line or port-a-cath?"

Grace says, "PICC lines are easy; they can be done by the nurse at the cancer clinic. The disadvantage is they hang out of your arm, they're cumbersome, they need weekly dressing changes, and you can't immerse them in water."

Rob's a bath man, I think. Losing baths would be huge.

Grace continues, and her tone tells me she's weighing it all, "If it was me and mine, I'd get the port-a-cath. But this would not be common in pancreatic cancer. But Rob," she looks directly at him, "if you continue on this trajectory that you're on, it's not unreasonable to think you've got several more cycles of chemotherapy ahead of you."

This is a significant statement. It's one thing for my mother to project more time for Rob, but quite another for Grace to say this. We are into our fifth round of chemotherapy. I wonder how many more she thinks he can receive — apparently enough to justify a port-a-cath. This is a concrete symbol of hope. We have more time, again.

"Let me see what I can do," says Grace.

She runs with the ball. She contacts Dr. Fryer, who negotiates surgery time in Woodstock Hospital, and the local surgeon. The surgeon is sceptical, but Dr. Fryer reassures him that Rob is doing very well. Normally, people with his condition don't live long enough to have shot veins, and, if they do, they usually receive PICC lines.

Within two weeks the surgery is scheduled and a go, for 8 February.

Rob's in bonus time. The port-a-cath will open a whole new horizon. We have options of more cycles of chemotherapy, and now the health care professionals are talking about months instead of weeks. Months means more time together. An answer to my prayer for more time.

"I'm still here," Rob keeps saying; "I'm not going anywhere." He is still here. It is amazing. He hasn't gone anywhere, yet.

Friday 29 January 2010
Rob Update

We've just come home from chemotherapy, Rob's second treatment of chemotherapy round six. I can't believe we've almost finished six rounds. The chemotherapy is generally going smoothly. The challenge after six rounds is that he has almost completely run out of usable veins in his arms and hands. We have systematically eliminated nurses that are able to successfully find a vein, and today, our favourite nurse Patrick even had trouble, taking forty-five minutes to get a line in, and needing to stick Rob twice before getting the IV started.

We had seen this coming a few weeks ago, so we started asking about options for venous access, and after some deliberation over whether to get a 'PICC line' or a 'port-a-cath', we have opted for the latter. A port-a-cath (for those who don't know) is a small plastic and silicone disk (size of a quarter but thicker) that leads to a long flexible plastic straw that goes into a vein.

Long story short though, Rob's having the surgery to insert the port-a-cath on Monday, February 8th, and it is nerve wracking no matter how great the end result may be. It seems however that we may not have much choice with the current state of his veins, as we still want to continue with the chemotherapy (since it's working so well), and it needs to go into a vein. So say a little extra prayer on the 8th!

Rob and I, the little kids, and my parents did get to Great Wolf Lodge in Niagara Falls a couple of weeks ago. It was wonderful. The kids had a great time, Rob went in a wave pool with the kids a few times, and we happily sat in deck chairs in the eighty-four degree inside temperature in our bathing suits and watched the kids swim and play and go down water slides.

We couldn't have done it without an extra set of adults, my parents were so helpful, and since they were there, Rob was able to sleep when he needed and nip back to the room for medication, etc. It was almost like being on a Southern holiday for a couple of days, and thankfully Rob felt really well and managed restaurant meals and everything. I hope the kids remember it as a fun time with him, I'm sure they will.

On the heels of our Great Wolf Lodge vacation we did unfortunately have the Norwalk virus hit our house; it ripped through the little kids, then me, then Rob, all within a forty-eight hour period, and just after Rob's chemotherapy last week. It was deadly, but brief, although it has taken Rob longer to recover fully than the rest of us. Luckily we have some of the most powerful anti-nausea medication on the planet in this house, so once the first wave had finished for Rob, we were able to dope him up sufficiently with anti-nausea drugs to allow him to keep his pain medication down. What a roller coaster of a few days that was!

Rob's youngest brother Howard and his wife Lynn have been visiting for the past four days and leave on Sunday. They arrived in Canada last Sunday, but we suggested they avoid our house until Tuesday to avoid the Norwalk bug, which didn't take much convincing after we gave them some detailed descriptions of the symptoms. It has been a nice visit, the second for Howard and Lynn, something we never thought would happen.

Rob's twin brother Malcolm and wife Caroline arrive on Sunday just as Howard and Lynn leave for a week visit. Again, another milestone we didn't think we'd see, a second visit from them as well.

We have had a few cards from people, which are so nice. The card parade slowed significantly after Christmas, as I think everyone had sent their best wishes throughout the fall and through the holidays, so it is nice when Rob gets the odd card. Thank you.

Rob continues to do so well, the little bumps along the way with stomach bugs and stubborn veins are part of it, but he continues to fight these little battles and win. And for now he's putting up a tremendous fight on the biggest battle. My dad came back from Florida with a bag of one hundred used golf balls in a sack. He handed them to Rob and told him he expected every one of them to get used, which Rob said he would.

Everyone on this distribution list knows how incredible Rob is and how strong and positive his spirit is. I'm sure those who come up with prognosis statistics didn't count on such strength of spirit and commitment to those around him. Please continue to keep Rob in your prayers and thoughts; it has worked wonders so far. At the beginning of this ordeal we were told three to six months. It will be six months on February tenth.

Take care

Keep the faith.

Jen

CHAPTER 11

Rob Days

⬭

Thursday 11 February 2010
E-mail from Monique to Jen and Rob

> *Hello Rob and Jen,*
> *Just wanted to give you guys a heads up on what we've been brewing here. We are organizing a fun fund-raising evening on your behalf, stag and doe style, with music, games, silent auction, etc. We are planning to host this event in the Norwich area. A planning committee has been set up and more information will be forthcoming. From you, we need to know the best possible time Rob would be able to make his presence to this event (which week in March would be ideal?). We are all very excited about planning this event and look forward to sharing laughter and fun times with you guys. Will keep you posted.*
> *Monique*

Friday 26 February 2010

Jen

"WOW! CAN YOU BELIEVE THIS?" Rob asks me in amazement, staring at the letter in my hand. He sounds excited, and maybe a bit overwhelmed.

We've just received the letter announcing his Sisters of St. Joseph's award. It's an honour we're both very aware of, having worked at Parkwood Hospital for years. I can remember receiving e-mails asking for nominees while I was there. The letter indicates that the ceremony will take place in the Parkwood auditorium and that each recipient will deliver a short acceptance speech. I'm so proud of him. Yikes, a speech!

"What should I wear?" Rob asks me, a hint of worry in his voice. This is no light question. I realize that any formal clothes in his closet will no longer fit him and that he will never wear them again.

"Well, I think we'll probably need to buy you some new dress pants and a dress shirt. I don't think you need to wear a jacket or tie or anything, but probably more dressy than a golf shirt," I say lightly, masking the stab of pain engulfing my heart.

The steroids and oedema have caused him to put on weight, both in his body and in his face. His weight gain is something that I barely see unless it reveals itself in the need for new clothes. One of my fears was that he would become skeletal — cachexia is the emaciation that accompanies later stages of some cancers. Rob's body has not succumbed to that. I'm so glad, yet I know his puffy cheeks and face cause him to be self-conscious in front of other people.

"We'll go shopping tomorrow and get you some new clothes, something that looks really nice, and that fits well," I say briskly, as if this is the simplest thing in the world.

"It seems like a waste of money to buy new clothes now," Rob says, sadness in his voice. I know where his mind is. He has lived seven months with this disease, which is longer than he 'should' have. He resists any purchases for himself, knowing he won't get much use out of them.

I lean over and kiss him. Even in this moment, when we're celebrating this award, there is always a reality check. He will not be here for much longer. We both know that. His mortality is always breathing down our necks, and it takes every ounce of will I have not to crumble in his arms and sob. Big breath.

"Well, OK, we won't buy you Hugo Boss, but we're going to buy you something nice. You can't go up in front of all those people in your shorts and T-shirt! Anyway, you have lots of dress shirts that you've probably only worn once or twice. This will be no different."

"OK." Rob agrees, "I'm your chubby hubby now!" He adds with a smile, "I wonder what my waist size is?" and pats his tummy, diverting the conversation away from his inevitable death. I smile, and hug him. How many of these hugs will I still have?

"You know, you're going to have to write a speech as well. It says so in the letter. Have you had any thoughts?"

"Mmm," he pauses. Rob is so understated — speeches are not his thing. He's not one to take the limelight with gusto. He grins at me again, "Maybe something like, 'Thank you, everyone'?"

"I think you're going to have to do a bit more than that! There will be a lot of people there who haven't seen you since you left work last July. They will be there just to see you, so I think you'll have to say a few words. And I think you should mention your diagnosis."

It's just becoming clear in my mind that this will be the first time Rob has been at Parkwood for more than a minute since his diagnosis. We went there back in October, to return his parking transponder. He was in and out in seconds. It had been hard for him to walk through the doors again, and he hadn't wanted to drop by the physiotherapy gym and see any of his colleagues. The weight of this award, and of the public ceremony at his beloved hospital, was starting to register. It would be a very emotional day. It would be a goodbye.

"Why would I mention that?" he says, looking puzzled.

"Well, it's the elephant in the room. And I believe you should always introduce the elephant in the room. You don't need to make that the focus of your speech, but I think you should mention it, somehow. It's an opportunity for you to personally say thank you for the support the Parkwood Hospital gang have provided, both in relation to your illness and the award," I encourage him.

"OK. I do want to say thank you. It's been incredible. The Parkwood family has been incredible." He says, decisively, "We'll work on the speech tomorrow."

Friday 26 February 2010
Phone Call from Jen to Helen

Helen

"HI, HELEN, IT'S JEN." Jen has called in the perfect moment, when I am without patients and not on the phone. This is happening regularly, it seems, in our interweaving of journeys.

"I was going to send you an e-mail about an award Rob's receiving, but I thought I'd pick up the phone instead! I know you worked at Parkwood Hospital once upon a time, so do you remember the Sisters of St. Joseph's awards?"

"Yes, I do remember. They're a huge honour to be nominated, as I remember."

"Well, Rob's been nominated and is receiving one! It will mean so much to him. A testament to his outstanding abilities in his profession, and as a person, I think."

"That's amazing, Jen. He so, so deserves it. How is he?"

"He's doing well, port-a-cath's in, without incident. We're heading to chemotherapy today. The port makes life so much easier. We're in a nice lull right now, and I'm trying to enjoy every minute of it. Friends and colleagues of Rob's from Parkwood have organized a fund-raiser for our family, 'Rob Day' is being held in mid-March at the community centre in Norwich. I don't know much about it — but again, another demonstration, I think, of how much Rob has touched so many lives and how people want to give back. It's mind boggling."

It amazes me as well. Life *is* showing up for them. "What an unexpected gift to come your way at this time, all this outpouring. I am so very glad he gets to see how well loved and honoured he is."

"Well, we have to get to chemotherapy. I just wanted to tell you the good news. I'll e-mail you the 'Rob Day' invitation."

"That's great, Jen. If I can be there I will. All the best."

We say our goodbyes.

How the unexpected gifts can find us.

Friday 26 February 2010
E-mail from Helen to Jen

Hi Jen,
Great, great poster for 'Rob Day'! Love the pictures; you are both
so alive, despite the struggle and heartache.
I don't think hope arising from your lived experience is false, Jen
as you asked. Is it false to believe that the body is wise and can, if not
heal, at least stave off the inevitable in amazing ways? Is it false to
believe that there is a great weaving happening through every single
thing in our lives that whether death finds us sooner or later, each
moment is part of something greater, the dreaming of this earth that
we all are part of? Maybe Rob has his own images of putting mind
to work on how his body can deal with those out of control cells with
his own images (medicine!).
Take care, Jen.
Helen

Friday 26 February 2010
E-mail from Jen to Helen

Hi,
Looking forward to seeing you after all of our March events. Rob
and I were talking this morning about the upcoming events and all of
the turns our life has taken. He says in contrast to his life before we met
that everything is so effortless now, just always seems to fall into place,
that's what we always used to say, can't exactly say that now, as this
cancer has been a mountain of a bump in our journey through life, but
we've learned a lot from this experience as well, and as always, we're
riding this wave … this choppy, nauseating wave, together.
A big change since I last connected to you is that Rob and I have
synchronized our bedtimes. He has started to be able to stay up a bit
later, and I, after months of refusing, have starting taking sleeping
pills a few times a week. It means I sleep. What a concept! And we get

to go to bed together like we always have. It's a time when I cry often but also feel such connection to Rob as I drift off next to him. Grace once again saves the day as she pushed me to use the sleeping pills. I think she likely picked up on my sleep deprived frazzle.
    Take care Helen,
    Jen

Saturday 27 February 2010
E-mail from Helen to Jen

Hi Jen,
    What a gift, sharing sleep has something deep to it. Grace can track your needs so artfully. I think sleep is one of the keys to resilience, along with good food. We forget that, I think. They seem so insignificant and beyond reach, eating and sleeping, when such huge emotionally challenging things are happening. And maybe sharing sleep strengthens that energetic bond we have with those we love and perhaps some wise part of us knows that love energy on the heartline is nourished by sharing sleep and dreams.
    So, all that to say, I am really glad and again I see the green shoots of life and wisdom pushing through the dark soil of this whole experience in your lives. It gives me hope that life does indeed never abandon us. Somehow it is wrapped around the kernel we call death and keeps breaking death open, like a seed, again and again into new life. May it continue to be so for you both every moment.
    The best to Rob. Your children stay close in my heart as well.
    Helen

Tuesday 2 March 2010
E-mail from Jen to Grace

Hi Grace,
    Looks like March is going to be a busy month. Anna Bluvol and

three other ladies from Parkwood Hospital arrived today to tell Rob of his nomination and winning of the sisters of St. Joseph's award for excellence. He was blown away and got teary.

Rob was selected for his excellence in his profession and focus on patient care, not as a gesture due to his present situation. That meant more to him than anything. The ceremony is at Parkwood Hospital on the nineteenth in the afternoon, so I'm sure many of his colleagues will be there to cheer him on, as will my parents. We went out this afternoon to get him some new dress pants and a shirt; he didn't have any that fit!

So, C.T. scan on the eighth, ROB DAY on the thirteenth, oncologist and chemotherapy on seventeenth, St. Joseph's award on the nineteenth, Jessica has a dance show in Waterloo on the twentieth, then the endocrinologist on the thirtieth and some more chemotherapy thrown in for good measure. Quite a month, hopefully he holds up.

Hope all is well Grace.

Jen

Tuesday 2 March 2010
Rob Update

We've had a really good last couple of weeks. Rob has had two chemotherapies in round seven through his new port-a-cath since I wrote last. He now has a one-inch scar, three inches below his collarbone and a small lump under the skin. Haley (my daughter) calls it "Robbie's on and off button"! It is the most wonderful device; I think we should all get one! The chemotherapy nurses at the cancer clinic are very adept at using 'ports', and Rob reports it is almost painless. What a change from having forty-five minutes of digging for veins using a needle!

In general Rob has been tolerating the chemotherapy very well the last several times. The cocktail of drugs that he is on continue to work, and he seems to bounce back from any minor side effects within a day or so. At his last oncologist appointment, the doctor seemed pleased, and indicated we'd just keep going with chemotherapy as long as things seemed to be working. So that's the plan, long may it continue.

Chemotherapy and the rest of the medication have certainly taken its toll. The biggest and most challenging new addition to the medication regime is insulin. Rob is now an insulin dependent diabetic. The doctors believe it is likely 'steroid induced hyperglycemia', which means it's brought on by long term steroid use (Rob takes steroids to control nausea and pain), but it could also be a result of the pancreas not producing insulin due to malignancy.

We don't know, we just know we have to stab Rob several times per day to measure blood sugar, and then several more times per day to inject insulin. I have the utmost respect for anyone who needs to master the art of blood sugar control, as it has been challenging to say the least.

Rob's medical team have unanimously reported to us that we are not aiming for perfect blood sugar control (thank goodness), as the long term implications of poor blood sugar control do not apply to Rob (i.e. we are not going to need to worry about Rob's circulation fifteen or twenty years from now because he will not be here). However, we do need to keep his sugars in a 'safe' range, for which he needs stabbing and insulin. So, less IV stabbing for chemotherapy, more fingers and tummy stabbing for diabetes, it's a trade-off I suppose! As you can all imagine, Rob NEVER complains about any of this, just keeps on going.

Rob decided a few weeks ago that maybe he might try and reduce some of the pain medication he's been taking for six months. He has been on quite a hefty dose (enough to sedate an elephant type doses), as the pain from pancreatic cancer is quite considerable. With the guidance of Dr. Fryer, he's now reduced his total daily dose by about twenty-five percent, which is quite an accomplishment seven months after diagnosis.

He says he's not done; he would like to keep trying reductions as long as he remains pain free, which he is at the moment, most of the time. The reduction in pain medication, and the tweaking of a few other medications, has meant that he's feeling more alert and 'himself,' something that friends and family have commented on recently when they have visited him. Rob continues to amaze us all with his determination.

The people on this distribution list have all received the invitation to 'ROB DAY' on March thirteenth. I don't even know what to write about this. Rob and I received an e-mail a few weeks ago giving us a 'heads up' that this event was in the works. We were and are flabbergasted. The organizers of this event are all high achieving, super organized, brilliant, caring, dear friends that Rob and I hold very, very close to our hearts. I don't know how to thank you girls!

We can't wait for ROB DAY. I know it will be so meaningful to see so many faces that we haven't seen since Rob was diagnosed and it will be wonderful to have a mix of family, friends, work colleagues, neighbours.

The amount of support that has continued to pour in from those that know and love Rob has been unwavering and quite overwhelming. Rob and I have commented to several people that we feel so humbled being the recipients of such an outpouring of support. Rob always says "I don't know what I've done to deserve this, I'm just me".

The support has been and I know it will continue to be one of the strongest forces that keep us going. It is almost like a collective 'will' that urges him to keep going, keep fighting, keep living to just stay with us. I'm sure it has something to do with the power of prayer, whatever your religious bent may be.

So, this brings me to our latest news which has happened just today. I've attached a picture of Rob and a few ladies taken just this morning in our living room. They arrived on our doorstep this morning to tell Rob that he had been nominated for, and selected as a recipient for this year's "Sisters of St. Joseph's Award for Excellence".

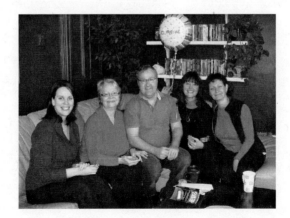

A committee of people nominated Rob and apparently interviewed several peers, patients and colleagues who have worked with Rob over the years. The nominations (which are apparently several pages long, with several sections) are 'blinded' and made anonymous, and then voted on by a committee.

I was told today that there was no mention of Rob's illness or present situation within the nomination, so this was not a 'gesture' made due to his cancer diagnosis; this was awarded based on his incredible gifts as a therapist, a colleague, a person. Rob was so surprised, he was truly speechless. "I'm just me" was all he could say when our guests left today.

The presentation of the award is March nineteenth, Parkwood auditorium, from two to four p.m. I hope we see some of you that day.

So, it's been an eventful few weeks, many positives, and many reasons to pause and celebrate what a great guy Rob is.

Rob has his second C.T. scan on March eighth, before Rob Day and the St Joseph's award ceremony. It's a nerve frazzling experience to go for a C.T. scan with this diagnosis. It's grown, stayed the same, or shrunk. We were so lucky, blessed last time as the tumours had shrunk. He surprised everyone with that. This time we're just hoping that they've stayed the same and not grown, not pushing our luck for more shrinkage. Mostly we're hoping Rob continues to feel well and enjoy all of those around him for as long as possible. That's what matters.

So, say a big prayer for a good C.T. scan and continued great symptom management and hopefully we'll see many of you on the thirteenth or the nineteenth.

Jen

Monday 8 March 2010
Another CT Scan

jen

WE'RE DRIVING INTO LONDON for Rob's CT scan. Rob is really quiet as I drive. The morning of a scan he can't eat, so he has an empty stomach other than the multiple pills he has to take each morning. I know he feels crummy.

I ask him, "What do you think the scan will say?" I've started to rely more heavily on what Rob thinks is going on inside his body.

He pauses for a bit. Then he says, "I don't think it's grown a whole bunch. I would think maybe it's the same as the last scan."

I ask him, "What makes you think it will be the same as the last time?"

He responds, laughing, "Well, I've had my Roombas working on it! I think they've kept things at bay."

I just accept this as a reality and hope that he's right. He's still here.

We go to the waiting room after Rob has consumed his four glasses of radioactive liquid, and a nurse enters to call him for the scan. Rob stands up to go, and he looks back at me, I look at him as the nurse glances at me and then says, "It's OK, you can come in with him."

This has never happened at any other scan before. *How close to death do you have to be before they allow your wife to come in with you? Did she read his chart?*

We go into the CT scan area, and a young, pregnant nurse appears. She says cheerily, "OK, Rob, we're going to start an IV line in you for the contrast dye."

I panic. Grace had warned us that they couldn't use the port-a-cath for CT-scan dye. I've no idea how anyone is going to find a vein. We've heard numerous times that his veins are shot. I warn the nurse of this. She looks a little nervous. After the third unsuccessful attempt she calls her supervisor. Eventually a different nurse appears, and after two more attempts she finally finds a vein. Thank God!

Rob does not flinch the whole time. He just takes it.

They wheel him away into the scanning room, and I wait just beyond its doors, listening and praying.

Monday 8 March 2010
E-mail from Jen to Grace

> *Hi Grace,*
> *Thanks so much for looking for the results for us; these scans are*

killers on the psyche, no matter how many good reasons there is to have one. I sat in the room today with Rob. Once he went through the double doors, I could hear the breathing instructions and the airplane taking off noises of the C.T. scanner, prayed harder and with more conviction in those five minutes than I have in a while and it dawned on me that there must be a lot of traffic back and forth to god, or whoever, from inside the walls of that hospital. Amazing how a few thousand computer images can change your life forever.

I'll be in touch, take care

Jen

Wednesday 10 March 2010
E-mail from Grace to Jen

Bottom line: There has been improvement since the last exam. Measurement is two point one by one point six centimeters (previously two point nine by two point four centimeters) of the pancreatic tail mass. There is no significant change to the liver.

All good, guys. Have great day!

Grace

Wednesday 10 March 2010
E-mail from Jen to Grace
(2½ minutes later!)

Wow! Thanks so much for the early update Grace. This is great, great news.

I look forward to talking with you about the report in more detail, but this is a fantastic and uplifting summary.

Many, many thanks for keeping your eyes out for this.

Jen

Thursday 11 March 2010
Rob Update

A quick update about Rob's C.T. scan results from Monday. Fantastic news! We heard yesterday morning that the C.T. scan showed the metastases in the liver showed no significant change, and the mass in the tail of the pancreas had shrunk further since the last C.T. scan in November.

We are, of course ecstatic, humbled, terribly relieved and so thankful. I personally found myself overwhelmed with emotion with the news, and sat in my car crying with thanks and gratitude after I dropped my kids off at school yesterday morning just after we found out.

Yesterday, when we received this news it was seven months from the day Rob was initially diagnosed (August tenth). A result like this makes you pause and reflect. I have written the statistics for this diagnosis many times before in these updates. We were initially told "several weeks to several months" and the literature widely quotes "three to six months" with a median survival of about five point two months when patients receive Gemcitabine chemotherapy for metastatic adenocarcinoma of the pancreas (which is Rob's treatment and diagnosis).

Clearly Rob is on the right side of the curve, and clearly Rob is still here for a reason. I can think of five very important reasons for him to still be here and we all live in this house. Rob is the rock that holds us all steady and the glue that ties our family together. People that know him personally know what a wonderful father he is and I can attest that he is a tremendously caring wonderful husband, with a deep ability to love and care for others.

Although Rob lives an ocean away from his family in England, we hear from them daily, and have been lucky to have so many visits. It is so clear how close Rob is to all of them, and how much strength he gains from them.

How fortunate we all are to have him with us and to be given this gift of time. So many people have been touched by Rob, personally and professionally. I know that many people said a silent prayer, or sent positive energy, or best wishes for continued good results. I'm so thankful to everyone who continues to keep us in their thoughts.

Our spiritual care provider, Helen, told us something in a session a while back that has really stuck with me, and that I've thought about a lot in the past twenty-four hours. I hope I don't misquote her. Helen has worked as a hospital chaplain in the past in palliative care and now works in spiritual care at the cancer clinic. She's wonderful. She also has, I think, a very, very difficult job, as many (most?) of the people she sees are facing death.

She told us that over the years, in her role as hospital chaplain, and also now at the cancer clinic, she has counseled numerous families in the final months, weeks, days and hours of a person's life on this earth. Helen says that the body has wisdom beyond what science or medicine can explain. She says that she has personally witnessed this time and again. The body's wisdom is at least partially responsible for when a person lets go and dies, and when they continue to live. People who are predicted to live three weeks live a year, and people who are predicted to live six months live three weeks. People hold on until their daughter flies in from California, or people slip away when the family breaks the bedside vigil and goes for coffee, the body has wisdom. Rob wants with every cell of his body to stay here with us and for the moment, he is.

On Monday I sat outside the C.T. suite, in the inner waiting room, while Rob was inside getting the scan. There were nurses, other patients, a coordinator, all sitting within ten feet of me but I found myself head bowed, hands clasped, tears streaming down my cheeks, almost begging for no tumour growth. I'm sure I was quite a sight. I'm also sure I'm not the first person to sit outside those double doors in that position.

So, for now, our prayers have been answered. Rob continues to defy the odds, he continues to feel reasonably well. We remain vigilant for any side effects or symptoms and do our best to keep them all at bay The sun is shining, the golf courses are melting and I'm sure he will make it out to play a round in the next several weeks.

Thank you to everyone who thinks of Rob and wishes him the best.

That's all for now

Jen

Saturday 13 March 2010
Rob Day

Jen

ROB IS SITTING in the kitchen with his coat and shoes on, waiting to go. I am scrambling to prepare Jack and Haley, and Ben and Jessica are getting ready as well. The house is a buzz of activity that we haven't seen in months.

"Well," I ask Rob, "are you ready for this? How are you feeling?"

He looks a little nervous and apprehensive. "I think I'm OK. I feel OK. The weather's really awful out. I wonder how many people will come."

I sense that he's nervous that not many will come, which would disappoint everyone who has put so much effort into it. I have no idea about numbers.

"I'm sure people will come. How many do you think will show up?" I ask, wondering what he really expects.

He replies cautiously, "Maybe twenty to thirty?"

I start mentally calculating how many I know for sure: my parents, aunts, uncles, my brother and his family, the organizers, and I quickly realize there will be more than twenty to thirty.

I say, "I think there'll be more than that. But we'll see."

He responds, bending his head slightly and shaking it in quiet amazement, "I just can't believe all this is happening for me."

We arrive at the community centre, and the organizers greet us and immediately adorn Rob with a plastic crown and a green feather boa! He looks priceless! Green is his favourite colour and the theme colour for the event. He laughs. Rob is always such a good sport. He knows no shame for a good laugh.

I look around the room and see balloons and maybe ten people there. I feel tightness in my chest and worry. Almost in answer, I suddenly hear a crowd coming in behind us and a group of about ten more people arriving. Everyone is hugging Rob, and he has a huge smile.

Within an hour, people have packed the hall, and more and more are streaming in. I've been milling around, away from Rob. We're both catching up with colleagues, relatives, and friends. I don't take my eyes off Rob.

Finally we meet up.

I hug him and give him a kiss, and the crowds disperse, as if knowing we need a minute to reconnect. Tears fill my eyes as I ask, "What do you think?"

"It's overwhelming," Rob replies, "I can't believe all the people that are here."

He quickly goes through a list and asks if I've seen them all. We lean in closely to even hear each other over the music and the celebration, and I realize he has been standing for over an hour and a half!

There must be at least a hundred people in the room. Everywhere I look, people are handing money over to the event organizers. Our friends hoped the event would attract financial support, since I too quit my job to be with Rob in his last months. With Rob's sick-leave pay and my not working, our family income had dropped by two-thirds since he was diagnosed.

"What are people saying to you?" I ask him curiously in a quiet moment at the back of the community centre.

"That they're praying for me, thinking about me, pulling for me." He pauses in awe and then adds, with a big smile, "There are a lot of people telling me how much they like me. How I've affected their lives. People have just been incredible." He pauses again.

I hug him tight; my eyes are welling with the tears always lurking. We're both feeling so many emotions.

"It's pretty overwhelming," he whispers quietly, allowing me to hold him close. "I keep thinking that people wouldn't normally get to experience this. Thoughts aren't usually shared like this unless it's at your funeral, and then you can't hear it because you're dead."

There's a rare catch in his voice. This has clearly moved him deeply. And here's the reality check in the room. I keep hugging him even tighter.

"Lucky me, I get to hear it!" He steps back and smiles at me with his big grin and lightens where we've landed … as always.

Monday 15 March 2010
Rob Update

It's taken Rob and me almost two full days to synthesize the events of Saturday, "Rob Fazakerley Day". We're finally sitting down to compose a thank you e-mail to all of the people who organized the event, attended, sent cards, bought tickets, and supported our family on Saturday. This is a bit like a thank you speech at the Oscars I think. We are filled with gratitude towards anyone who was in any way involved. I know that a lot, a huge, amount of effort went into this day and I'm sure we'll never know the half of it.

What a phenomenal day. Rob and I couldn't in our wildest dreams imagine an event like this. So many people attended, well over a hundred I think. The weather on Saturday was dreadful but despite this and the long journeys some people took to get there, I found the atmosphere in our little Norwich Community Centre amazing, the support and love in the room was palpable.

The afternoon seemed to fly by. Every time I looked at the door more people were streaming in. We saw people from all corners of our life. Colleagues and friends from Rob's work and my work, colleagues that haven't worked with Rob for years but wanted to support him, friends from public school and university, family, family of co-workers, neighbours, friends of our children, teachers from their schools, even the mayor.

And all these people made their way over to Rob to wish him all the best, to tell him how much he's meant to them, to say hello and tell him they miss him at work, to tell him they're praying for him, and to give him the clear message to keep up the fight because he is important to every person in the room.

So, I'm a bit lost for words as to how to thank so many people for creating a day that has given us such a message. Tonight as I was making supper, Rob and I were talking about Saturday (as we have been for a straight forty-eight hours now, save a few for sleeping).

After rolling the day around in my head for two days, I have decided that a couple of things have really struck me. At the beginning of this journey, way back in the middle of August, I sat at this same computer looking up survival statistics for pancreatic cancer five days after Rob was diagnosed. A grim task for anyone.

It was late at night, Rob was long in bed, and all the kids were either out or asleep in bed. I walked ten feet from our computer into our living room, dropped to my knees and begged someone above to give me time with Rob. I cried and felt utterly alone and helpless facing this terrible prognosis and impending loss of my true love.

Shortly after that we started receiving all the wonderful cards people have sent. So many had messages of hope, prayer, best wishes, and positive thoughts. I stood in the community centre on Saturday, and realized that so many of the people who have sent such meaningful words to us over these past months were there in the room, surrounding Rob and I, and holding us up. What a feeling. I can't describe it but it made me realize that we are most certainly not alone on this journey. We have so many people on it with us willing Rob to stay in the here and now.

In the early days I often questioned, and Rob and I discussed, whether it would be better to meet the end in a sudden event, a car crash for instance or to succumb over a prolonged period to a terminal illness. I'm not sure there's a right answer to that question. It is terribly, terribly difficult to watch someone you love fight something like this and know that eventually they will succumb to it.

I also know that very few people in this life get to experience so many people telling them how important they are to so many, to feel the love and support of so many and to realize how many lives they have touched. Rob has had that experience. That experience is thanks to so many people sending cards, and e-mails, and phone calls, and visiting us, and letting us know they care, and supporting us through an event like Rob Day.

So, thank you to everyone involved, from the bottom of our hearts. Thank you for organizing it (thank you to the husbands of those that organized it!), thank you for coming, thank you for buying tickets, thank you for giving us a magical, once in a lifetime experience of having so many people in one space channel so much good will.

Thank you to everyone
Jen and Rob

Monday 15 March 2010
E-mail from Grace to Jen

Hi Jen,
  It was an honour to be at Rob Day. The love in that building was palpable. I hope he had a good birthday on Sunday. Would have been a hard act to follow after Saturday's celebration!
  There was a mass of people and it felt alive with multi generations. Laughter, life, it was all about community. It was great to meet your family, Jen, and Ben and Jessica and your friend Julia with her new baby and also to share this time with our mutual colleagues, Anna and Donna. How much nicer it was to meet here rather than at Rob's funeral.
  Rob was "just Rob", demure, less than comfortable in the limelight. He spoke eloquently, from the heart in quiet humble gratitude. Rob never strikes me as someone who likes to do a lot of public speaking or have a lot of attention put on him but he spoke quietly, sincerely, eloquently and succinctly.
  I saw you and Rob milling and I noticed that you were quietly guiding Rob to sit and eat. He discreetly checked his blood sugar and took his insulin, on top of the details of his care as always.
  Such an outpouring. People from twenty years of his life and from all over Ontario. Great day!
  Hope you are out and about enjoying this glorious day!
  Grace

Wednesday 17 March 2010
E-mail from Jen to Helen

Hi Helen,
  I'm sitting outside on a lawn chair in the sun. Rob is inside on a teleconference with Parkwood Hospital about program restructuring in the stroke program. The director asked if he would mind participating via teleconference in a focus group. He's so excited to be engaged a little in work that he loved so much. So great to see.

I was thinking about my kids today. My kids were very little: one and a half and two and a half when I met Rob. I was so cautious and hesitant to bring him fully into my life at first because I felt I couldn't risk 'dating' someone who wouldn't be there for them long term. As I write that it seems strange because he in fact won't be with us 'long term', but I wouldn't exchange these years for anything.

But that's not what I mean. I didn't want my kids to have to live through another relationship breakdown. So it took a lot of soul searching before I 'let him in.' I know I wouldn't have if I had sensed any level of uncertainty. I think as women, and as mothers we have a very heightened sense of protecting our children from any undue emotional harm or duress, one of the things I struggle with most right now, as I'd love our kids to not have to go through this but Rob's situation is sadly not preventable. I just need to shepherd them through.

Talk soon Helen,

Jen

Wednesday 17 March 2010
E-mail from Helen to Jen

Hi Jen,

Yes, our children come first and foremost. We cannot prevent life's tragedies affecting them, as you are living right now and it is sobering that, despite your best instincts as a mother to prevent a loss for your children in your second relationship with Rob, life has come along and confronted them with that potential reality anyway. Ultimately, you name it so accurately, we cannot prevent them from encountering deep suffering, we can only 'shepherd' them through it.

I am very glad Rob day was such a gift to you. I know it will have given your children a deep, visceral experience of that 'grace' that seems so abstract in the midst of heartache and will be a touchstone for them, on some level, when greater agonies hit them, and you.

Ever in my heart and prayers.

Helen

Monday 22 March 2010
Rob Update

I've been sending lots of e-mails lately. We've had so many events happen that I want to include people in and thank people for.

As far as a health update, Rob is in the middle of his eighth round of chemotherapy. Our latest medical challenge is the ongoing struggle to try and reduce his dosage of steroids. Steroids are wonderful but carry with them a huge number of side effects, so we have been trying to slowly wean Rob down a bit, as the general rule of thumb is 'lowest possible dose'. Anyway, this is a challenge as the weaning procedure carries its own set of side effects including mild nausea and 'vague' pain which is extremely difficult to watch, let alone experience.

The main reason I am writing this e-mail is to provide an update on Rob's "Sister's of St. Joseph's Award" which he received at Parkwood Hospital last Friday.

The ceremony was just two days after Rob had chemotherapy so he was showing some of the physical effects of the chemotherapy (mostly puffiness which happens a couple days after chemotherapy) but the energy and emotion of the day kept him going. The awards ceremony was lovely with a choir singing and speeches from the CEO of the London Hospitals, as well as a board member and one of the current Sisters of St. Joseph's.

Each recipient of the award (there were six in total) was introduced by a member of their respective nomination committees with a short speech and then each recipient gave a speech as well. Prior to the ceremony, pictures of each recipient were displayed at the side of the auditorium, with a bound copy of each nomination. The nomination had several excerpts from interviews done with patients, co-workers, supervisors, colleagues, etc., all of which highlighted the exceptional qualities of each recipient. These 'testimonials' are incredible to read, none of which would surprise anyone on this list, they're all about how wonderful Rob is, how client focused, caring, team oriented, professional, kind, funny, all Rob.

My parents came to the ceremony to support Rob, as did (I think) the entire rehab team, who lined the walls of the auditorium until Rob spoke, then they all quietly left; it was very clear who they were there to see!

I have asked Anna Bluvol's permission to share her speech in this up-date e-mail. Anna has worked with Rob at Parkwood Hospital for many years, and is also a good friend. Anna was very involved in the nomination process. This will be good to read for those who were there as well as those who weren't there.

When Anna took the podium in front of the audience, her voice cracked and she had tears in her eyes. That was it for me, I couldn't hold back the tears and I don't know if there were many other dry eyes in the room. I heard a lot of sniffling and I know I missed many parts of her speech as a result.

So, here is what Anna said:

"Dear Rob

"On behalf of the entire rehab program I am honored and privileged to have the opportunity to speak from the heart. It is impossible to express what you mean and represent to us in the time allotted. When we put the call out for this nomination, tons of stories poured in: all exemplifying your compassion, empathy, sincerity, your gentle and caring nature and your exceptional sense of respect as a team player. Those of us who were fortunate to work with you side by side can attest to your unwavering pro-fessionalism and patient focus. We could always count on your honesty, yet the incredible ability to give hope to those devastated by their injuries and considered 'hopeless'; somehow you were always able to help them realize their goals.

"Rob, you are a superb, gifted clinician with vast expertise and passion about your work. You always amazed us by making things look so easy. Your natural talent to inject humor into your work, at patiently teaching and mentoring others make you stand out above the rest.

"As Jen previously said, you have the deep ability to love and care for others. You have always given from the heart, going above and beyond. You have touched so many lives, both personally and professionally. I am looking around the room and seeing so many people who are here to sup-port and honor you. This is a true testament of who you are and I hope you can sense and feel our love, support and respect! You have truly been an inspiration to us! And in all of this, you have never sought recognition, always so humble, wondering why all the fuss, thinking 'this is just me' — just being Rob.

"A huge thank you goes out to the selection committee for recognizing Rob's achievements. Rob, thank you from the bottom of our hearts for giving us the opportunity to honor you and celebrate with you! Thank you for being YOU! Congratulations!"

Rob followed with a short speech as well. He worked on it the day before and delivered it so well. The audience gave a long standing ovation after Anna's speech before he spoke, and then again after he spoke, it was so overwhelming to stand in the crowd as his wife and partner.

I was so incredibly proud of him and felt surrounded by a room full of people that recognized all the incredible traits that he possesses. I felt so, so lucky to be married to him, and so grateful that he had been recognized like this by his peers.

So, here is what Rob said:

"Thank you so much. I came to Parkwood Hospital in 1987 as an 'imported' physiotherapist from England. With the exception of a couple years in the middle I have worked my entire professional career in this hospital. Over the years I've worked on teams in Stroke, Spinal Cord Injury, Acquired Brain Injury and most recently on the Community Stroke Rehabilitation Team.

"I have always seen my role as being part of a team and I've always loved my work. So, it is overwhelming to be recognized for excellence as an individual and for simply doing what I love, which is providing patient care.

"This award is particularly overwhelming at this time, as seven months ago I was diagnosed with metastatic pancreatic cancer. To be recognized at this time means so much more.

"My career at Parkwood has always meant so much to me. Parkwood Hospital is like a family, and over the past seven months the support for my family and I has been unbelievable. It's an honour to be recognized by my peers for my professional achievements. Thanks to everyone involved in the nomination process. Thanks to all the teams I've worked with these past twenty-three years."

Rob thanked the nomination committee and I would like to as well. This e-mail won't convey the feeling in the room last Friday for those who weren't there but I wanted to include as many people as I could in this incredible event. Juxtaposed against the previous Saturday, "Rob Day," it felt very different. It was more emotional, there were a lot of tears.

It was hard for Rob to walk back through the doors of Parkwood Hospital. He hadn't been there since before his diagnosis and it was an act charged with emotion. Rob saw many, many people he hadn't seen since before he was sick and so many people hugged him, shook his hand and wished him well. I've said this before but to have people recognize you for what and who you are when you are still 'here' is a wonderful gift. I'm so appreciative of everyone involved who took the time to recognize Rob for the wonderful person he is and honour him with the award.

On a personal note, I also had many people come up and thank me for these update e-mails, both at "Rob Day" and at the awards ceremony. These updates mean (I think) as much or more to me writing them as they do for those who receive them. For me it is a reminder of what is going on in the 'here and now'. It is so easy to let your mind travel forward in time to a place that is very sad but these updates keep me focused on the facts, many of which are positive, in Rob's current treatment.

More importantly, though, these updates for me keep people engaged in what's happening with Rob and make sure that he stays in the front of people's thoughts. If the past seven months have shown me anything it's that I am not alone in thinking that Rob is an extraordinary, precious person who needs to stay here with us for as long as he comfortably can and I want these updates to serve as a way of making sure that nobody forgets about him and how great he is. I don't think anyone ever will.

So thanks again everyone for continuing to support Rob in this journey.

And thank you as always for keeping him in your thoughts and prayers.

Jen

Reflections: Winter 2010

Jen

I REALIZE LOOKING BACK that a shift happened around Christmas. I handed over living in the darkness of the imminent threat that Rob was going to die any day and reached the place of saying, "I don't know how much time we're going to have, but we're going to *live* this." We stopped putting timelines on things.

In the beginning we hoped to reach Christmas. After that event, and Rob was still living and comparatively well, we just hoped for 'Don't go,' or 'Just stay,' or 'Long may this continue.' We didn't artificially put any timelines on it. We realized that aiming for Christmas put us in a strange predicament after December 25. Suddenly there was no Christmas anymore between us and Rob's dying, and I realized it had been a way of staving off the inevitable.

I knew there was no way that we were going to master this cancer or control it. We knew it was going to win; we just had to sit back and let things unfold and do everything we could. 'Everything we could' meant we bore down into the lived experience of it. It didn't mean that we just relaxed. There was a huge amount of clinical juggling during this time between the medical team and Rob and me to make sure his symptoms were under as much control as possible. Looking back, I realize how well we did this and how very complicated it all was. It was different than at the beginning.

I would have regretted it deeply had I not done all that I did, trying to master the knowledge and all the tricks that everyone gave us — doctors, Grace, spiritual care. I read a lot, downloaded a ton of information into my brain, made sure we were doing every single thing possible — not to fight the inevitable but to gain more time and quality time, when we wouldn't need to chase symptoms constantly. I was trying to make sure that we were doing everything possible, and then we could relax into the experience of being together, living now.

It was, as I said above, like changing from a sprint to a marathon. The first part was trying to obtain all the information, do everything we could.

We'd gained knowledge, and, even though we never believed the cancer would not take his life, we stopped feeling as if it was going to eat him alive, as we had at the beginning. It was the feeling of 'bonus time.' We didn't want to waste this precious time, so there was a letting go, a shift into the new year and the new place we were in.

And, of course, along came, seemingly out of the blue, the wonderful Rob Days in March, which my guy was healthy enough to savour to the full. They reminded us of all the love and support and solicitude that buoy our spirits and help keep Rob and me going.

Part Four

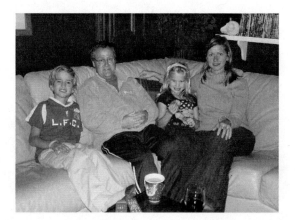

Spring 2010

CHAPTER 12

Come Dance with Me

∽

Friday 26 March 2010
Fourth Spiritual Care Session

Helen

ROB IS SITTING in front of me. Jen is next to him on the couch. None of us expected to still be meeting almost seven months from our first session, let alone talking about hope. Last September we were in Gethsemane, wishing deeply someone or something would take this cup away from Rob. Yet here we are, all these months later, in the living experience of hope.

They wanted to come and tell me about the month's events, especially Rob Day and the Sisters of St. Joseph's Award.

"The day of the ceremony, at least a hundred attended, and many were there for Rob," Jen tells me. Their eyes are so bright and shining with life. Rob, in his quiet way, radiates with the fulness of this experience. This amazing gift from 'life' came along to give his spirit buoyancy and something huge to focus on for all the weeks prior. Now, after sharing their news about it, they are feeling its afterglow. Their cup is running over with gratitude and joy. It is striking and moving.

Jen continues, "The walls were filled with staff that came from the hospital floors, and people lined up out of the door to shake his hand and congratulate him."

I remember that auditorium from working there. It is a very large space, and I could picture it overflowing. I think how this experience is giving Rob an incredible mirror of who he has been in his life, reflecting his essence, his care, his skill, and how many lives he's touched so quietly, so invisibly, now reflecting back to him in full force. Nothing discreet or invisible about this moment. Life's given Rob centre stage. I wonder what that is like for him.

Jen says with a touch of awe, "Most people don't get this until their funeral, when they can't hear it." She goes on to describe Rob in his work. Her love and respect for him are manifest. Once again, I notice the tremendous bond of deep, deep love, almost like a palpable energy that brings more light into the room. It happens every time.

She continues, "He always loved to work with the ones who seemed hopeless to everyone else. He could get people walking that were never expected to walk again. He loved to work with the worst kind of strokes and had amazing successes. He'd just go over, talk quietly, touch them gently, and, next thing, they're half way across the room!"

Rob just sits, present, and he clearly has become the master of his skills and gifts but has no need to talk about it. 'Humble' is the word that comes to mind. Genuine humility. What a rare quality.

Jen laughingly says, "Years ago, I had the privilege of seeing Rob in rounds sometimes. When the physicians wanted to move someone on or not admit them because they seemed so hopeless for rehabilitation, Rob would take them on and say, 'But there's always potential.' And they'd look at him like he was crazy but give the patient a chance because it was Rob saying it. And Rob always had great results."

An even greater respect is arising as I hear about Rob at work — a gem in the physiotherapy room whom I didn't know at all as I was walking the corridors in a different part of the hospital. How many worlds within worlds there are!

"Rob, I wonder where such an innate sense of possibility comes from? What or who in your life has created that movement towards 'possibility' in the most impossible situations?"

My tingling intuition is telling me that here was perhaps a clue as to how a man who has received only a very short time to live is still here with us, so remarkably and relatively stable.

"I don't know really," Rob replies quietly. "I can't think of any person like that in my life. It's just always been there."

Again, that 'just is-ness' about who he is. I continually feel like I am revolving around a Zen koan, a paradox. How can he have such an impact on people, including me, when he understates every aspect of who he is? It's just so rare to meet someone so very present to himself, to others, and to the 'what is' of his life and not need anyone to hear, see, or recognize him for it.

I think of the statement I heard once, "The enlightened one walks into the room, and everyone feels change, but no one knows who or what caused it." An effect Rob seems to have.

As I look at him and think of the months of walking alongside him and Jen in this grappling with life right in the jaws of death, I think of how he has just stayed present, so present to the whole experience without overt resistance, without clinging to what was and is no longer, without bitterness or even anger, simply here, simply with his beloved, simply being in the whole experience.

As I've come to know him in his unassuming manner, I suspect this is how he has lived his whole life. 'We die how we live' seems very true to me in this moment, as it has in many moments of witnessing in my work, but for opposite reasons.

I see Rob and Jen's deep love, their absolute commitment to the 'real' of their experience and their diagnosis, their unwavering remembering and acceptance of its fatality, while they experience an incredible wellspring of life, love, and being that I've never before witnessed in people facing the guillotine of death. They have miraculously managed to wrench themselves away from the magnetic gaze of death, like deer in the headlights, that paralyses so many people when cancer lands in their lives.

Over and over they have turned to living and grasping life with both hands in every moment possible. It has been agony so many moments. Jen has described the times of keening that overwhelm her. Rob, in his own quiet way, faces the horror from within his inner landscape. His heart tears open as their young children decorate the Christmas tree and he knows he may not see another Christmas. Unusually, his tears spill over into visibility, yet celebrate the day they did, with gusto.

And they have been living this way for the last seven months. Curiously, within this unwilling 'school of living in the present moment,' the horizon of death has kept unexpectedly receding. First the metastases in his liver shrank, and then his pancreatic tumours! His body seems to be metabolizing the cancer, working with the chemotherapy and medical support, and all of it together is claiming life, cell by cell, prolonging it against the odds.

My intuition is sensing that this is not at all about cure — that something else is happening here. A metabolizing of something cellular, in the depths of the energy that Rob is, that we all are, that will arc across death and grows stronger to do so through this time of their love's deepening, strengthening, solidifying. Somehow this process has to do with shaping their future beyond death.

As I listen to Jen describe Rob's work, the interplay of hope and hopelessness he feels for people 'deemed hopeless' strikes me. His capacity to stir the potential in individuals with a stroke or a brain injury and create with them a story of hope that they inscribe in their body against all odds moves me. And now, here he is, doing it with cancer in his own life and for his love, Jen. He hasn't stopped fostering hope, believing in the possible in the crucible of the impossible, and gaining time that seemed unimaginable in September.

What a tremendous gift he is and that he is giving by his lack of resistance to dying and his full and complete embracing of life — 'enlightenment,' for once, does not seem an overstatement. Yet, so without any need in him to think that of himself. It's tremendously refreshing and powerful.

Jen continues her stories about him, "There was a woman who had suffered a stroke and seemed to have no chance of walking ever again, and she was assigned to Rob. He went to her bed and encouraged her to sit up and try to walk with him. She excused herself with various reasons and kept brushing him off, and so, finally, Rob held out his hand and said in his lovely Scouse accent and charming smile, 'Come dance with me!' And she did. She actually took his hand, made it out of bed, and let him hold her to help her rock on her feet like in a dance. This was the beginning of her recovery."

We all laugh. What a moment.

"What a metaphor for how you're living this experience with cancer, Rob," I respond. "It's as if life has offered its hand to you in the midst of dealing a pancreatic cancer in your body and said in your own words, 'Come dance with me.' Against the odds, you've chosen to take up the offer and dance with no holding back and dance hard, no matter how short your time may be. It's really incredible."

He looks at me with his steady gaze, hearing my words and nodding. Somehow, I am the one experiencing affirmation — in my hope that surely we can stare death down and let it challenge us to live as we never have before. And to follow Rob's example and just take up life and live it to the full.

There is clearly no lying down to die here. Living is the business at hand, and this is exactly what Rob and Jen are doing, because of their deep and real river of love, which flows continually between them and around their children.

The power of love. Here it is, right here in my office. The privilege of my work overwhelms me in this moment. Who has a chance to witness such depths, such 'real,' at the very heart of life?

"You are a living example of alchemy," I reflect to them, "where psychic energy streams together between people and creates something 'new.' You are two lives drawn together by a bond or 'something,' as you described it, and it has formed into a powerful, alchemical love, transforming both of your lives and your children's.

"You have become a holon, an ecosystem that is bigger than the sum of its individual parts, that has drawn hundreds of others into its field, creating a field of energy among us all that is bigger than that of the cancer. Yes, the chemotherapy has good results for a short time, extending life, statistically, but this cancer can take many a strong person down so very quickly."

We all know the likely end of this story. But in this moment, life is clearly showing up, and my instincts tell me that this will somehow change their experience of his death.

I can see Rob's eyes again, like in our first visit, holding my gaze deeply, taking in every word. Somehow it feels as if he is pulling these words out of me with the part of him that knows this instinctively, willing me to share these words with him and, perhaps more particularly, with Jen. I realize with a new clarity that he's quietly teaching her. He's quietly doing this, showing Jen in his own life now what he's shown others in his care for them, and I am giving the language. Rob is gently guiding Jen to places he has intuitively trusted all along.

I continue, moving with some inner current, "We watch the crocuses emerge in spring and miss that they are teaching us about life and death, revealing the truth that life always shows up, one way or another. That it may not come in the way we want it to, that we may not be able to avoid loss or death, the same way a seed cannot avoid 'dying' to become the flower, or the flower cannot avoid 'dying' to become the seed, but life always re-emerges one way or another, the green shoots push through concrete.

"The descent of loss is terrible. There is no avoiding its agony or heart-ache. But if we remember the wisdom of the snowdrops and learn to see the signs of life showing up at our door, we can hold ourselves in the agony, knowing that it's only a matter of time and life will find its way through once again."

Life has shown up for them, creating wave after wave of love that finds its way in, through, and towards them, in the midst of the agony. I feel the living presence of what I am trying to 'language' with these words in the room. Life *has* shown up.

"I see in you, Rob, the tremendous courage to take what life has dealt and still take life's hand and dance with everything you've got in every moment that you're given. And Jen is right there with you in the dance. The full force of her powerful love that you sparked within her is poured out, her cup running over for you. Love is revealed as 'presence' that creates life and transforms everything — even death."

"Yes, that's how it feels," says Jen. "That's exactly how it feels."

Rob nods his agreement.

"Well, we need to go to chemotherapy" — Jen notices the time.

Heartfelt hugs. We are in mutual awe of what we are in together.

Rob says, as they're leaving the quietness of my office, mimicking Monty Python, "And now for something completely different." We laugh. So true.

"We leave your beautiful sanctuary and go out into that 'other' world," Jen comments wrily. "It's always so jarring to leave here and face the busy-ness and entirely different feel of the clinics."

I wish for the millionth time for a more holistic health care system where what we have just experienced — this type of thing happens behind many closed doors of all kinds of front-line workers' offices — could become an integral part of the care of each and every person, if they wished for it. How different cancer care might be!

They leave, and I sit down and take a breath.

Today I have witnessed and been a part of the alchemy of the true meaning of hope right here in my quiet, hidden room within our cancer program building, which, to many observers, seems a battlefield. In this moment, in my room, rather than witnessing a battle, I have seen the strength and fierceness of a tango with cancer. A fiery dance with death, with Jen and Rob looking it square in the eyes, not burying their heads from its presence, but choosing to dance hard with everything they've got. This tango with death is creating so much life in and through them that I find myself weeping for the awe of it. What a privilege indeed to bear witness to this with them.

This moment together has been a living experience of words such as 'faith,' 'hope,' and 'sacred.' And there is no need to speak those words. They simply resonate through the experience of this courageous couple who keep choosing to dance in love and life, even if this moment is the only one they have.

And is this not how we would all do well to live?

Friday 26 March 2010
E-mail from Jen to Helen

> *It was great to see you, Helen. I need to let you know that I felt very 'hopeful' when we left you today. Felt that you mirrored what I've been seeing in Rob, that he isn't ready to go, so he isn't. I have to admit, it's not a feeling I often am left with at the cancer program, and everybody's a bit too factual and statistical at times. So thank you for giving us that, not false hope, just affirmation of something I've been witnessing.*

Late at night when I curl up next to him, often teary because my tired mind takes me to a time when I won't be afforded such a presence in my bed, I'll say "Just stay," and if he's awake, he always says "I am." So present.
Talk soon,
Jen

Thursday 15 April 2010
Rob Update

It's been an incredible month of milestones. One more milestone yet to come is one that involves some hope. We have rented a cottage for the end of June beginning of July to try and squeeze out one last (or maybe not) summer holiday for our family. One of the most difficult things that Rob and I have faced with this disease is the inability to plan anything for our futures, because there may not be one. We started talking about renting a cottage on the lake last summer, actually just when Rob started to become visibly ill but before anyone knew other than us and before we knew what was wrong.

We decided after the last C.T. scan that we should go ahead and rent it anyway and luckily we were still able to secure it for a week (Craig, if you are reading this, thanks). It's the first thing we've planned that is so far in the future and the practical side of me also made sure it was wheel chair accessible, and reasonably close to the cancer clinic. Anyway, we're all really looking forward to it and I know we'll get there.

I think that's all for now. Rob's feeling good, more chemotherapy to come. Thanks to everyone as always for their continued unwavering support. The support of our family and friends is absolutely as important as any medication and chemotherapy in keeping Rob as well as he is. So please keep sending all those positive thoughts and prayers, because I know they are working.

Thanks,
Jen

Monday 3 May 2010
E-mail from Jen to Helen

Hi Helen,
A funny thing about spring flowers, we've always had a lot of forget-me-nots scattered throughout the gardens around our house. Rob says they're his favourites. Last summer, I said out loud to Rob that I knew I'd always think about him when I saw forget-me-nots and I hoped they would come back again.

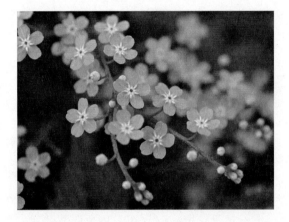

So this year, we have a bumper crop, maybe five times more than before and there was nothing we did differently last year to them. I have thought more than once, that if I didn't have Rob here with me this spring, the tons of forget-me-nots would have been saying something to me. I guess they are anyway.
Just sending you a picture of them in our backyard, just went out and took it before I rouse the kids for their day. What a beautiful day today.
Take care,
Jen

Thursday 6 May 2010
Rob Update

Rob and I have been enjoying the beautiful spring weather, and have had a fairly quiet few weeks since my last update. On the treatment front, Rob has finished his ninth round of chemotherapy. Each "round" consists of 3 chemo treatments, once a week for three weeks in a row, then a week off to let the body rest. He was scheduled for his third treatment of round nine last Friday, and unfortunately his chemotherapy was deferred for the first time since he started chemotherapy last September.

Upon arriving to chemotherapy each week, Rob has blood work done to check his blood counts, and ensure that he has enough of each type of blood cell to withstand the assault of chemotherapy. Gemcitabine (the chemotherapy drug) is apparently quite hard on platelets, and sure enough, this last Friday Rob's platelet count was too low to proceed.

Chemotherapy is of course designed to kill or disrupt cancer cells, but unfortunately the collateral damage is that the therapy also kills other cells, bone marrow cells in this case (which produce blood cells). We have been warned that we may be 'deferred' due to 'low counts' many times and amazingly Rob's bone marrow has somehow managed to be hardy enough to sustain all the treatments without a problem. But, as we are reminded of continuously at the cancer clinic, chemotherapy is cumulative, and over time the bone marrow becomes 'tired' or damaged, and needs a rest to regenerate.

So, we left the cancer clinic a little low on Friday having not received this life sustainer. However, as we always seem to do, we had the whole thing rationalized within a couple of hours, "if the chemotherapy is killing the bone marrow cells then hopefully it must be also killing the cancer cells", that "it must have been meant to be so that Rob could enjoy the great weather last weekend without feeling the 'hangover'", that "chemotherapy has a long half-life, so there would still be lots in his system fighting off the tumours", etc., etc.

Situations like this force you to live one day at a time, because you can't do a thing about them. From the cancer clinic we went over to the mall on Friday, we picked up a re-sized wedding ring for Rob (his fingers are a bit swollen on occasion, and we didn't think a finger amputation resulting from a tight ring would help his cancer any), and ordered him a new pair of eye glasses, as his old ones were several years old, and he had just broken them (for the second time) putting on a motorcycle helmet (story to follow below). Spending money on sizing a wedding ring and new glasses is our way of reassuring ourselves that Rob will be around long enough to need and enjoy such things.

On another positive note, we had some nice weather last weekend, and went on a 'date' to Port Dover on Saturday after the treatment deferral. We wandered around shops and had a meal, it was wonderful, and something we normally wouldn't be able to do on a Saturday after chemotherapy.

Since my last update Rob has played two games of golf; nine holes each game with my dad at the local golf course (small course, using a golf cart, but still great). Rob recently received a 'Big Bertha' from my dad, who found it second hand in a golf store in Florida on their recent trip there. A Big Bertha is a fancy golf club, a driver, which Rob has really enjoyed getting to know. His game has improved since diagnoses. I wouldn't recommend it as a strategy, but it's nice to see him enjoying the game.

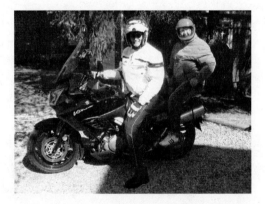

So, the motorcycle story. Benj, a good friend and colleague of Rob's recently bought himself a motorcycle. He dropped by to see Rob last week again, but this time on his new bike. Towards the end of the visit he offered to take Rob for a spin, which Rob was thrilled about. I was out of the house picking the kids up from school, but apparently when Rob put the spare helmet on, his glasses snapped right in the middle.

They carried on, rode around some country roads for half an hour or so, and came back. I was home by then and heard the bike rumble in the driveway. Rob was perched on the back behind Benj. Now Benj is very tall (around six and a half feet) and Rob is most definitely not! The motorcycle is designed for a tall person, so Rob needed a little help from me to pull him off the bike, but what a big smile.

As I re-read what I've just written it sounds like a very relaxed life. We are really, Rob's diagnosis has forced us to live one day at a time, and really LIVE while we can. I said to Rob recently as we were sitting out in the sun on a Tuesday afternoon, I likely won't have a retirement with him, so in a way it's nice to enjoy one with him now.

In the beginning of all this, it seemed like a sprint. We had to race to get a diagnosis, a treatment plan, pain and symptom management, medications sorted out, wills written, last wishes sorted, and we all grieved very intensely and painfully at what we thought was just in front of us.

It has now gone from a sprint to a marathon, and the pace seems so different. We had to go through all of what we did in the beginning to get where we are now, but in a way it now seems like it's time to just sit back and enjoy each other and our family. We have a full house again as Jessica is now back from university for the summer and there seems to be a lot of life here in the house.

Recently I've found myself trying to describe the support we have received from all of our friends and families to various people; our CCAC Case Manager at her routine re-check, Dr. Fryer, Grace, our nurse practitioner, friends, etc. I have been trying to convey the message that it's not just the chemotherapy and the supportive care medicine that has kept Rob going, it's his spirit, and his spirit is sustained by the support of everyone around us who have continued to provide the practical and emotional support these past nine months. Our case manager called it the wind beneath his wings, which is a bit corny, but bang on.

So thank you everyone once again for all the support, the ongoing cards, emails, best wishes and prayers. They have and will continue to sustain us on this marathon.

Many thanks,

Jen

CHAPTER 13

Tipping Point?

⚭

Friday 4 June 2010
Rob Update

We've had several e-mails and phone calls asking how Rob's doing, usually an indication I'm due to write one of these. We've had a mixed last few weeks. It is likely, based on two deferrals of chemotherapy to allow Rob's platelets (which allow his blood to clot) to recover, that Rob will be put on a 'chemotherapy holiday' where he has no treatments for several weeks, in the hopes that his bone marrow can regenerate and grow strong enough again to handle the assault of more treatments.

We've heard all along that this drug is particularly hard on platelets, which it is now proving to be. The risk of this is of course that in the absence of chemotherapy, the cancer will gain strength and start to grow again. This is worrying to all of us. However, bone marrow is pretty essential in the grand scheme of things and it appears that we will be forced to change treatment in some way, at least for a while to let it (hopefully) regenerate.

So, if anyone needs something extra to add to their prayer list, or a thought to attach to their good wishes, no cancer growth and lots of bone marrow regeneration and platelets would be great! (Not sure if it all works like that, but it's worth a shot.)

The interesting thing about low platelets is you feel fine. Rob's subjective health is quite good right now. He remains pain free most of the time, has a good appetite, sleeps well, has a great outlook on life, and in short bursts has some energy. He has been out to play golf several times with my dad, usually once a week, and has even tried a few new golf courses in the area. He plays with a cart, and does nine holes, which takes him two hours and results in him being pretty tired the rest of the day, but very satisfied. He tells me his golf game has improved significantly, a game he only started playing last spring. People on this list know how extremely positive Rob is, so perhaps this statement is no surprise, but he told me the other day how lucky he was to have this time off so he could improve his golf game.

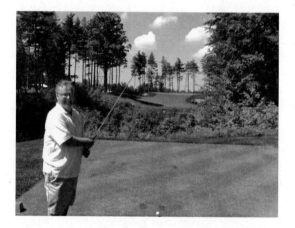

We've been spending lots of time in our backyard enjoying the weather. Rob has a significant golfer's tan, despite lots of sunscreen (chemotherapy makes skin very photosensitive), and has developed very curly hair in the last couple of months, again likely a side effect of the chemotherapy.

So, some worrying news about bone marrow and platelets, some good news about 'feeling good' and playing golf. This is our life right now. This potential break in chemotherapy is the first significant change in Rob's treatment plan since September and it's very easy to let our minds go down a path where this change may represent a tipping point or a change in tack.

We are constantly reminded about how well Rob is doing, how his survival to this point has far exceeded expectations, and I always think to myself when I hear doctors remind us of that: *Well of course! He is extraordinary.* He always exceeds expectations. Rob's motto, whether in his personal or his professional life has always boiled down to two principles: everyone has potential, and every challenge is an opportunity. So, we're trying to see this bone marrow hiccup as just that; a hiccup that we will somehow overcome together with a lot of prayers and best wishes, and clinical expertise holding us up.

The belief that everyone has potential is an interesting one. It has not been lost on either of us that being given the diagnosis of metastatic pancreatic cancer is like being given a message with no potential. A short prognosis comes with this diagnosis, and a zero percent chance of survival. Yet Rob has kept going, and I think I can say he has truly enjoyed the time he's had since his diagnosis. He doesn't feel sorry for himself and often in a day we'll have conversations about how lucky we are to have this time to spend with each other, with our children, with Rob's family in England, with friends. Rob often says he feels lucky. Pretty amazing.

Rob insists this will not be a tipping point, he's not ready to go there yet; things to do, golf to play. And that is what I think faith really means, it's putting aside the worries and future dread and listening to someone's will to keep going, and believing that he'll somehow do it, with lots of help, and just enjoying what you've got today.

I think that's it for now.

Jen

Sunday 13 June 2010
E-mail from Jen to Helen

> *Hi Helen,*
>
> *I'm lying on the couch, Rob asleep and kids with their dad, very quiet, reading "Love, Medicine, and Miracles" by Bernie Siegel. This is an older book written in 1986, author is a surgeon and is describing the "exceptional patient"; strong will power, engaged in recovery and in life. It's really interesting and I'm finding it very relevant. He quotes Jungian therapists frequently and it makes me think of so many of the things you've said.*
>
> *We met with the oncologist Thursday, and after a discussion (which*

was exceedingly long for him) we've decided to defer chemotherapy for a cycle to "save some chemotherapy for later". He said Rob will only be able to have a certain amount in total and that we need to think of the future and it's good to have some in our back pocket for use when he's very sick, that a break as opposed to a series of one off deferrals would be less likely to trigger resistance in the cancer, that his bone marrow will be able to recover more if there's a break and allow for more concentrated future chemotherapy.

He said if he were a betting man, he guessed Rob would be exactly the same in a month at our follow up visit. So this is when I really need to put my trust in medicine and hope we've made the right decision, hope the cancer doesn't see this opportunity to grab hold again. I asked the doctor what he would do knowing he is young, married and had a young child. He looked uncomfortable, and then said he'd take a break. So be it.

Anyway, a painful and difficult decision, but I think we've made it and are at peace with the decision.

Now more than ever Rob has set to work to keep this disease at bay. I said to him last night that I think he has old energy of a healer in his hands. He has healed so many people who were said to be 'broken', he always sets his goals higher than other therapists as far as what he believes he can achieve with patients and more often than not achieves the goals. I asked him to turn whatever that ability is onto himself, which I suppose he's already done, but a good time now to up the ante.

Thinking of you lots, Helen, and all your words of wisdom.
Jen

Sunday 13 June 2010
E-mail from Helen to Jen

Hi Jen,
*   Love how the books are finding you as you need them. That's an example of the dreamtime, weaving many things together but in the*

same 'theme', it's the medicine finding you. Belief is one thing, past experience is one thing, but we need real time ongoing experiences, breadcrumbs from life, to keep affirming us on our path through the dark, difficult forests.

Tough decision, yes. It affirms once again my statement to many people that even though you have the guidance of the doctors, in the end, you still need that 'bone deep wisdom' of your own gut to make decisions. I take the tough discernments to my sleep and ask for clarity. Often I'll wake up with the 'knowing.' I need a gut peacefulness of rightness to a particular choice. It's the sense of one thing leading to another, always.

So, if you've made peace with this moment of choice making, one thing will lead to another and you can trust that whatever happens, your bones have guided you on the path which are deeply connected to the ever shifting, weaving, life making web we are all integrally embedded in.

This physical form is so compelling to us, especially in western society where we really have no other realm open to us in our minds. Yet, it is but one aspect of multi-dimensional realities. All this to say, I have no doubt, that whatever happens, this web of weaving that has been so amazing thus far, will continue to hold you. It will continue to weave gifts and patterns through the weft and warp of the heartbreaking struggle of this experience.

You are definitely not alone in this whole journey. And I will add my prayers, as always, that Rob's body continues to metabolize this cancer in powerful ways; that of course is always the hope; if I were to put money on anyone staying stable without the chemotherapy I'm putting it on Rob!

A thought in this chemotherapy respite, ask yourselves 'what medicines do I want to fill this month with?' Keep doing what you've been doing and maybe Rob can ask his wise heart-mind what this month can be filled with. What would be good medicine for him? So rather than feeling like something isn't being done i.e. chemotherapy and 'waiting', turn it around into a both/and, so that the chemotherapy is being temporarily replaced with different kinds of medicines *guided by Rob's heart-mind each and every day. Ask yourselves, as you have all along, what is the 'medicine' I need today? Go with the energies, trust whatever comes and do it.*

Jen, I'm not sure you see how profound your own journey is through this but, trust me, you are living this in one of the most deeply courageous ways I've ever witnessed. You are living the zen koan of cancer: "Keep one eye on death while the other eye is on living; keep one eye on meaninglessness and the other one on mean-ing-making," the proverbial 'eye of the needle'. Not many manage that, often landing one side or the other of the koan and clinging to it. While you cling with all your might to the hope of Rob's living a miracle, you still keep one eye on what I hear you name as 'reality' with a clarity of seeing that is so painful for your heart, but nonethe-less, wise.

Have an ease-filled day. Holding you very deeply in this 'knife edge, present moment living' you are in and living so, so amazingly. It is ever a privilege to walk with you both in this pathless path.

Helen

Monday 14 June 2010
E-mail from Jen to Helen

Hi Helen,

You always seem to e-mail me when I need it. I know it shouldn't matter, but the faith in you and the oncologist, and Grace, all 'betting' that Rob will remain stable for the month wells me up with a feeling of calm. I feel like this; I feel like he'll be ok, that it's not his time to deteriorate, that his shoulders are strong, that he can do it and it's reassuring to hear others also think that. So thank you for putting that into your e-mail. We're offered so little hope to hang on to, but sentences like that provide me with a bit of hope.

We're heading out for a walk in between storm clouds, the birds are all 'twitter-pated' talking to us. What a commentary on our lives!

Jen

Reflections: Spring 2010

Jen

GRADUALLY, IN WINTER AND SPRING, we shifted from hoping for a 'thing' or event in the future to living in the moment. People kept asking us about our thoughts on Rob's prognosis, and they'd say, "Wow, isn't it amazing that he's still living, and maybe he'll be the one that beats the odds and live." We didn't let that suck us in. We always knew and faced the reality that this would kill him. Rob would always answer those questions or comments with, "Oh, I'm not done yet," or "We've decided our new goal is that we're aiming for chronic disease!" or "We'll just take it as it comes."

By spring, we were at the top of the parabola curve — there was quality of life, fun stuff with the family, and it always felt as if we were on a teeter-totter and just balancing on this tip. It was 'Don't look at this side into the future, or that side to the past.' Keep the symptoms under good control, and go a little bit into the future so you can keep the symptoms under control but not so far that you go into his dying. I would force myself to stop looking too far ahead. I knew it was temporary, this place, and it was no plateau.

And the break in chemotherapy starting in May brought a new and unexpected shift in gears. We always had to be watching for trends and markers and planning for the next chemotherapy or CT scan. That was mostly my task. I would always be watching for decline. We balanced it with Rob's unbelievable level of calm and acceptance and his attitude of "Well, life's terminal! We'll take it as it comes."

We knew a decline was coming, so there was nothing we could do about it when that happened, and it seemed senseless to waste time focusing on the fact that in the future it would be worse. It was the huge gift that Rob gave me that he always had this equanimity about his own mortality. That made it possible for me to live each day with him, alongside him. I took that on as my role, along with doing my very best to make sure he was not suffering with acute symptoms in any way. It was beyond a full-time job, it was huge. This then allowed him the quality of life and to hit golf balls in the back yard, and, because he could, we focused on our quality of life together every single day.

I think because we knew he had so little time it made it seem wasteful to spend our days in worry. I know Rob thought a lot about how difficult it was going to be for everyone when he died and how we'd cope with the loss. He talked about how much he was going to miss everybody, but then he'd add, "So, I'm so glad I'm here now." I remember his sitting on the couch and saying, "I wish I didn't have this cancer. I wish I didn't have to die and leave you all. But I can't change any of that, so I'll just enjoy the time I've got." He always had an answer for the angst that came with the reality we were living.

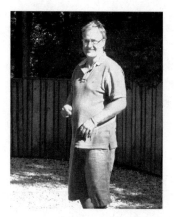

I was banking my time with him. I would consciously ask him all the questions I thought I'd want to ask him in the future. Knick-knacks in the house from England, their stories, movies he loved, his dreams for the kids, how things worked in the basement that I knew nothing about. I realized he was well enough to have all these conversations, some of them quite frivolous, but all with both of us well aware that there would come a time when he would not be there to ask.

Every day was a deposit in my bank account of memory for the future.

Part Five

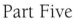

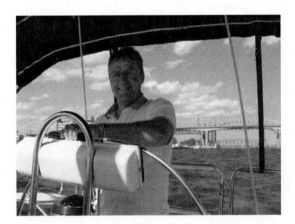

Summer 2010

That which hurries towards the rising is small,
that which approaches the descent is great.

− C.G. Jung, *The Red Book*

CHAPTER 14

A Week at the Cottage

∞

Friday 25 June 2010
E-mail from Jen to Helen

Hi Helen,
    Rob's had a few days that were less than great in spots, had a bit more pain (he's been almost pain free for months on the same dose of pain meds) that had me wracked with tears last night, facing this cancer again that we've managed to have a little break from the bull's-eye.
    The bull's-eye refocuses very fast as soon as he's not feeling well. The pain he gets is intermittent, and in between he seems great, makes the roller coaster effects more intense. Last night while I was blubbering away stroking his hair, and saying how this period with no chemotherapy felt so isolating, with so little direction on 'when to start back to chemotherapy' (in my mind I'm saying 'today? He's had pain, its growing, do we go back with chemotherapy?'). He said he'd know when it was time to go back to chemotherapy, that the longer he stays off, the less chance for resistance, the more chance for bone marrow to grow (all true) and he seemed so calm saying it, he said he wasn't going anywhere. So, we slept.
    Rob's almost done reading Bernie Siegel's book. I think it's really spoken truths to him, I've never seen him read so keenly.
    Tomorrow we head to the lake to stay at the cottage for a week

with our family, all the kids (Ben for only some); my parents, my brother and his family live five minutes away. Everyone's looking forward to it so much. I never thought last August we'd be gearing up for a family holiday almost a year later. Thought I'd be putting flowers on tombstones.

Rob is so exceptional; I hope he can keep going. This part of the journey has brought us so close we're almost one and the same, it's palpable. I know he's not feeling well long before he tells me. If I'm in the next room, doesn't matter, I know. I knew yesterday and it was so scary.

"Let it Be" by the Beatles always plays in my head when I've had a big cry or when I worry about a medical decision, like last night.

Take care, Helen.

Jen

Monday 28 June 2010
E-mail from Helen to Jen

Hi Jen,

Know that I hold you both, as always, and appreciate the 'specifics' while you're at the cottage.

I have this belief that somehow it's not about avoiding the 'roller coaster,' just about living it fully, trusting the momentum will always bring you somewhere different, somewhere new no matter whether 'this moment' is an 'up' or a 'down.' Perhaps for a more organic image, it's being in the waves that life is, washing us somewhere different every time. Best not to struggle against them, be in them, as you are. In the end, it is all the same ocean, death, life, joy, sorrow, pain, healing. All the same 'life', just looks different depending on where we are in the 'wave' of the moment and you are living it, profoundly, deeply, acutely, agonizingly and with incredible spirit.

I believe Rob will know when to start back on chemotherapy. His bones are trustworthy in their knowing.

My great care to you both,
Helen

Wednesday 30 June 2010

Jen

I CAN'T BELIEVE WE'VE MADE IT to the cottage. It was a monumental task. Of course, Rob couldn't help with the packing like in the past. It seems to have taken ages, so much contingency planning for every medical possibility. We have a whole bag full of medications, not the normal cottage packing.

The last two nights Rob has not slept well. I'm trying to decide if it's different surroundings and activity level, or the different bed, or if something else is going on. I have an ominous, dark foreboding feeling that this is not just a side effect of the new environment. I start mentally calculating the extra breakthrough pain medications Rob's taken in the last twenty-four hours, and I lose count. At least three or four more doses per day. I've already given him extra this morning, and it's only eight o'clock. I'll e-mail Grace and ask for advice.

I hear Rob stirring in the bedroom and go in.

"How are you doing, sweetheart?" I ask him. I look at him lying in the bed in this very small bedroom in the cottage. The place is small and spare and has furniture from the 1970s. It's right on the beach; the view of the crystal-blue Lake Huron reaching to the horizon is breathtaking. Rob's eyes meet mine. I can tell he's in pain still.

"I think I probably need another breakthrough," he says.

"No problem," I respond, already taking the pill out of the bottle. I help Rob sit up and realize that in the last two days he seems to need more help getting out of bed. I try to convince myself that I am imagining this or that the bed is different from ours at home. Yet the strain on my back tells a different story. He's worsening. Something has changed.

Rob swallows his pill and looks at me. I see worry in his eyes.

He says, "I think I've been taking a lot more breakthrough, haven't I? I've got a lot more pain. I don't know if I should be taking this much breakthrough."

I take a deep breath. Here it is.

I force my voice to remain calm, "Have you noticed anything else different?"

He says, "I can't get comfortable when I sleep. I just feel so tired."

In my mind, I calculate how many weeks he's been without chemotherapy and what I know about how fast this cancer can grow. I try to step back and look objectively at him: his abdomen looks bigger; he looks like he's carrying more fluid in his hands and feet. I realize, reviewing the last two days, his appetite has changed. He also looks grey.

"Well, Rob, there are no heroics in this game. If you have pain, then we treat the pain. There is no 'I should' or 'I shouldn't.' There's lots of reason why you might be experiencing more pain here — you're in a different bed, different location, and different levels of activity, different food, and a long car ride, and as we both well know you're on a chemotherapy holiday and I suppose this cancer is probably growing. And that's not going to be a surprise to either of us.

"I'm going to connect with Grace this morning and come up with a plan. We've managed your pain and symptoms so far, this whole time, and there's no reason we can't do it now. We just have to tweak a few things. We're here at the cottage. We've got our family around us. We never thought we'd get here. We'll make this work." I am reassuring myself as much as him.

Rob leans over and kisses me. "I know we will. I love you."

I tuck him back into bed, hoping he can sleep for a couple more hours, and close the door behind me. I stand in the kitchen looking out over the lake, tears streaming down my face. In my gut I know that this is not because of the car ride, or a different bed. This is the predicted re-emergence of this disease, and I know in that moment we don't have long now. Bonus time is over.

I wipe away my tears and grab my BlackBerry. I e-mail Grace a detailed description of the past seventy-two hours of Rob's symptom changes. I outline each additional dose of medication and hope that she responds quickly. I do not describe how my heart is breaking. How does one describe that? Easier to focus on the medical details, the tweaking.

Five minutes later, Grace responds and provides me with a plan to adjust the cocktail of drugs and, we hope, turn things around for the rest of our vacation. Grace has pulled another gift out of her bag of tricks. We can do something about this. I feel immense relief.

Wednesday 30 June 2010

Grace

I'VE JUST RECEIVED an e-mail from Jen at the cottage. I had an inkling things are changing, and it concerned me that they were heading to the lake and a different environment. What a great thing we can keep communicating by BlackBerry — I can support them and control his pain.

The end-of-life process is coming more quickly than we were hoping. What a monumental task Jen's just getting them all to the cottage. I feel some concern for her about this week at the cottage with Rob's subtle declining. I know she's more than capable of handling things but hope the toll isn't too great.

I've told her we can call in prescriptions to any pharmacy near the cottage and reminded her that the cancer clinic is only an hour away. I believe so firmly that there's always a lot we can do. Jen wanted to have all the troops there, and it's my job to support that. And where there is a will, there is always a way. They made it there anyway.

Pulling something out of the bag over and over chasing symptoms is intensely personal for me. Growing up as a farm girl you have to make things work. You have resources only to make do. The world of oncology reinforced this — people come in with dastardly diagnoses, but we still do things to make them feel better. I keep finding something to give Rob, some new tweaking that keeps those symptoms in check. But for how long, in this moment now, I'm not sure. I think the change is happening.

Wednesday 30 June 2010

Jen

GRACE'S TWEAKS WORK, once again. She's amazing. During the rest of our vacation, Rob's symptoms improve, but I know the beast is back. The decline has begun.

That night I have a dream. *I dream about a hurricane on the lake that is approaching, and I'm the only one seeing it, trying to get everyone to safety. Twice it approaches, and twice it just turns into rain. Eventually it disappears off into the distance.*

The next night at the cottage I am in bed trying to sleep. Rob is sleeping next to me. I keep seeing the hurricane. It is looming and threatening. It really upsets me. I'm no expert in dream analysis, but I feel in my gut that the hurricane is the cancer. I can't shut it out of my mind.

I decide to try some of the visualizing techniques we've learned from Helen and in Bernie Siegel's books. I try to imagine what could dissolve the hurricane. In my mind, I mould it with my hands as if it were red clay on a potter's wheel. Amazingly, it dissolves, and I sleep. The next night it doesn't come back.

Sunday 4 July 2010

Jen

THE REST OF THE HOLIDAY is everything we've hoped for. We spend every day at the beach, all of us lined up on beach towels. The kids swim and play Frisbee in the water. Rob and I even get out for a boat ride with my colleague Craig, who has rented the cottage to us. Rob plays a game of golf with my Dad and brother, and it's apparently one of his best this year. Big deposits in our memory bank for the future, which is feeling closer now than ever.

Friday 9 July 2010
Rob Update

We have had a very busy month and a holiday from chemotherapy. It is very nerve wracking to do such a thing. Chemotherapy is what has kept this cancer at bay for eleven months, so very scary to remove it no matter how strong the argument. Rob and I have been told numerous times that pancreatic adenocarcinoma is an aggressive cancer, kills people quickly, so the worry was that Rob would decline in the month off.

We saw the oncologist yesterday for the one month check after the chemotherapy break. Rob is basically the same as he was a month ago. Some small subtle changes in blood work, but nothing too alarming, and generally he is feeling all right. Rob's energy is still quite good, his pain is reasonably well controlled, and appetite ok, still playing golf weekly, and our family got away to the cottage for a week. He has good days and not so good days, and sometimes parts of his good days are not perfect, but in general we're still enjoying our 'early retirement' together.

Based on all of this, and the arguments for breaking from chemotherapy above, Rob has chosen to extend his break by another four weeks. We will see the oncologist again after this next break and re-evaluate again, but basically we are taking things month by month, and hoping things in the tumour department just stay quiet for the time being.

It was much easier this time to make the decision. I suppose because nothing drastic happened last month in the absence of chemotherapy. The oncologist was in full support of the decision to continue the break, but he's good as he leaves the decision up to Rob. He just gives the facts we need to help us in the decision-making.

So, we did get to the cottage with the whole family. My brother and his family live just ten minutes away from the cottage, so we saw lots of them, and the cousins all got lots of time together. It was a wonderful holiday. So many flashbacks to last summer when Rob was diagnosed, one of the hardest things we faced together was our inability to plan a future filled with family holidays, kids' birthdays together, Christmas.

Yet there we all were, together as a family, enjoying our time together. It all felt extremely normal, just a holiday at the cottage, sunsets over the beach, sandcastles, swimming, boat rides, campfires, a golf game for Rob; just what you'd expect. It was great to have my parents there, who helped with meals, looking after Jack and Haley, grocery shopping, everything. We couldn't have done this holiday without them.

It was also so great that Ben and Jessica both managed to get time off work and join all of us. They each brought friends; we set up a tent outside the cottage to make enough room for everyone. It was very festive!

Rob did so well! The overnight bag that the two of us used to share if we were going away for a night was full of medication, so that was a bit different, but we managed really well, and our family has a whole new batch of memories. I've attached a couple pictures.

So, that's been our month. Next month will also be busy. We're expecting Rob's parents for another visit towards the end of August for three weeks and I'm sure if Rob's up to it we'll do some little day trips together. We will start to prepare for Jessica to move back to University, living in a house this year with friends instead of Residence, so a big move to plan for.

We WILL celebrate Rob's first year since diagnosis anniversary on August tenth. Something we never thought he'd see, but I have every confidence that he will. We will all continue to revel in Rob's unshakeable will to stay here with us and his determination to enjoy each day. He is amazing.

That's all for now.

Jen

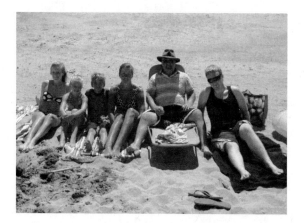

CHAPTER 15

The Descent Begins

Thursday 15 July 2010
E-mail from Jen to Helen

Hi Helen,

Rob is showing some signs of disease progression, which I suppose we were to expect in the absence of chemotherapy. His pain has escalated significantly in the past three weeks and really a lot in the past week. As of tomorrow morning we will have doubled his pain medication since three weeks ago, a hard pill (s) to swallow. I've found myself looking for alternate explanations, could this be anything other than disease progression but my mind knows I'm grasping at straws. We might request a C.T. scan and then we'll know, but I think I do already.

Rob is still optimistic; he says he feels that things aren't much bigger if at all. I wonder if he's just saying this for me. This is when I sing "let it be" in my head and try and listen to the lyrics. We have an option to see the palliative care doc first thing tomorrow morning in Woodstock if he's worse, if not have an appointment booked for Monday morning to see her here at the house.

Rob's groggy with all the additional breakthrough drugs he's been taking, but still in good spirits, not much can dampen that. He's not up to sitting in your office however, so we'll need to cancel tomorrow.

I'm so glad we got to the cottage. This all started there and got worse the week after. I think he staved it off as best he could for our holiday. And he did really, looking at what's happening now.

The palliative care doctor said the chemotherapy was still working at last dose, so it still should when he goes back. It's a balance game now, hoping he's recovered enough platelets to take some more chemotherapy. And of course hoping the chemotherapy will still work.

I think Helen you must have seen a million couples (ok, maybe hundreds? tens?) approach this same cliff face of disease progression after 'remission' (dare we call it that). It is so different than the initial illness and diagnosis. Seems more deadened, less laden with acute emotion and more real and solid. Like we've walked this road before, we're better prepared for symptoms, more educated about what every twinge means on a cellular as well as a treatment level. But it makes it very hard and sort of tender at the same time, like maybe this is it, and the last time was just practice. What a crappy thing to have to practice for.

I hope this finds you before tomorrow.

Take care Helen

Jen

Tuesday 20 July 2010
E-mail from Jen to Helen

Hi Helen,

I wanted to send you this latest update on Rob.

I have a funny story. I've been reading more Bernie Siegel, lots about dreams, expressing emotion, etc. About a week ago Rob yelled (quietly) during his sleep. Scared the #@! out of me. I woke him to see if he was ok, he smiled and said "I was just scoring a try in rugby", so just a dream. In a year that's the only dream he's ever told me about, he says he doesn't ever remember dreams. I've never ever heard him dream about rugby.*

Anyway, thought nothing of the dream until last night. A passage in the book I'm reading talked about a man with stomach cancer that had a dream that he was going to explode and the medicine he needed was like a bomb. Under some sort of therapy this man and his therapist came to the conclusion that he had to shout and yell, that was the bomb, something he had never ever done. (He must have been English). He went on to live many more years with this newfound ability to express all emotions.

Anyway, this intrigued me. I turned to Rob and asked when the last time he really yelled was, he said probably when he was twenty-two playing rugby.

Here's the funny part. We were alone in the house; I said, "Well, why don't you yell right now?" You would think I had asked him to streak naked through the streets of Norwich!! "I can't, it's Sunday. It would be weird." So lots of back and forth discussion, ending with me running up to the attic of our house, closing the door and screaming at top volume for ten seconds. When I came down and noted no police had gathered at our door, Rob relented, went upstairs to the attic by himself, and behind closed doors shouted loudly, twice! He came downstairs hungry and energized and said it was really weird. I think I'll encourage him to do it often.

So, shout therapy!

Hope you enjoy your time away from work.

Jen

Friday 23 July 2010
E-mail from Helen to Jen

Hi Jen,

I am laughing my head off at the thought of Rob, the quintessential Englishman shouting in his attic. It's perfect!

Great idea Jen. The synchronicities are abounding, I love it.

Helen

Friday 23 July 2010
Rob Update

Rob suggested that I do an update now, to bring everyone up to speed with how he is.

Some of our close friends and families have been kept up to date with what's been happening, but we realize the rest of the 'fan club' hasn't. We also realize this is how inaccurate information gets around, so we thought the group should hear from us directly.

We've had a very rough few weeks. Rob's pain started to escalate about three weeks ago, just before we went to the cottage. When patients start using lots and lots of 'breakthrough' pills, it means the long acting is not doing its job well enough getting rid of the pain.

Anyway, long story short, under the guidance of Rob's palliative care doctor we've gradually increased the long acting dose over the past few weeks and he now seems to be close to being relatively pain free or at least well controlled. In the end, the dose we've landed on (for now) is more than double that he was on three weeks ago and more than he was ever on. The palliative care doctor also doubled his steroids, another weapon in the 'pain' arsenal, which seems to have also helped a lot. Chipmunk cheeks times two!

Obviously, the increase in drugs has taken its toll. Fatigue and sluggishness are definitely more pronounced with the increased pain meds. Although we're hoping that Rob will accommodate to the new dose (which he's already starting to do) and perk up a bit. The increased steroids cause an increase in blood sugar, which means insulin adjustments. Not to mention the havoc all this causes on the GI (gastrointestinal) system. It's never just a simple med change; it's a bit more like a dominoes game. Rob in his typical Rob way, says that this is "all a bit of a nuisance", you know cancer pain, medication side effects, the lot. What a guy.

Despite this being categorized as "a bit of a nuisance" by Rob, I'm sure you can imagine this is extremely worrying for both of us. Pain was the only symptom that presented itself last summer when Rob was diagnosed and here it was again; same location, same type, similar intensity. This coupled with the fact that Rob is currently on a chemotherapy break has had both of us very worried that this was a sign of rapid disease progression in the absence of chemotherapy.

Scary stuff. Both our nurse practitioner Grace and our palliative care doctor have tried to be encouraging that this very well may not be progression, but just the lack of chemotherapy. Rob is with them. He thinks it's the lack of chemotherapy and its wonderful properties, and assures me he's not going anywhere. So there it is, just a nuisance.

If Rob's cancer shows more signs of progressing, then it's time to talk about chemotherapy again, and hope that his bone marrow can withstand it some more. This is no easy decision, and it's made a thousand times worse because nobody can tell us what the best thing to do is.

Very, very few pancreatic cancer patients are where Rob is almost a year after diagnosis. Most are soundly below ground and so there isn't lots of research supporting how best to proceed. The oncologist can't rely on his knowledge of the last ten patients who were in Rob's situation because there aren't any. Rob is unique, in more ways than one.

This last few weeks has certainly reminded us how quickly things can change, and how important it is for us to enjoy what time we have together when Rob is feeling well. Rob still has lots of things he wants to do and this has strengthened our resolve to seize the good days and do them.

These last few weeks has also made me realize how much we benefit from the support of those around us. Our families have been wonderful. Rob's parents call daily, and his brothers all call regularly. We're looking forward to another visit from Rob's mom and dad in August. My parents have spent the last week while Rob wasn't great having Jack and Haley at their house entertaining them as grandparents do, trying to give them a good summer. We continue to have cards and emails of well wishes and support coming in from across the globe, something that has been unwavering for Rob this past year. People will never know how much the cards and letters mean to Rob and me.

As usual, a dip in health forces us to focus our attention on all things spiritual, how and where we fit in to this world, how lucky we are to have one another and how to use Rob's incredible will and fighting spirit to keep him here with us.

I think that's it for now. I hope that this email inspires people to please send positive thoughts and prayers Rob's way. We may be entering a different stage in this journey and it's one that we will need much support for. Rob and I are forever grateful and humbled by the support that has been shown so far. So much of it being completely invisible to us, but we know it's there. Please keep it coming!!

Thanks all,

Jen

Thursday 5 August 2010
Rob Update

We met with the oncologist yesterday, and Rob will be starting back to chemotherapy tomorrow (Friday). During our appointment Rob said he didn't think he could wait any longer to start chemotherapy, and so we will try again. The oncologist was in support of this, and indicated that there was no denying that this was disease progression, and that hopefully Rob's bone marrow will have recovered enough to accept more chemotherapy.

We asked if a C.T. scan would be necessary, and were told "only if you want to know what you're up against. The C.T. scan would not have good news at this point, and the results won't help me make any clinical decisions". So, we have no need for the C.T. scan. Rob knows what's going on without one. We have been warned to fully expect not to be able to get many chemotherapy treatments before Rob's platelet count (or other blood cell counts) dip again preventing chemotherapy, but we're hoping and praying he can get a few to help with symptoms.

Once he can't have any more chemotherapy (and we're approaching that day), the options for palliation shrink, and this journey takes a different course. The chemotherapy will apparently take a cycle or two (so three to six treatments) before it helps Rob feel better (if it works), just as it did last fall.

This is a hard email to write. It's the first one in a long time (maybe the first yet) that we can definitively say the cancer has gotten worse and that's hard news to deliver and to hear. So, decision made; back to chemotherapy tomorrow after eleven weeks off. Rob is pleased to be going back and also pleased that he was able to stay off for as long as he did to hopefully allow his marrow to rebuild. The hope is that with the tumour not seeing the chemotherapy for a while it will be more sensitive to it, and hopefully respond well.

At this stage (as always) the focus is very much on symptom control to try and decrease pain and nausea and hopefully Rob to 'feel better', not on curing this cancer, or shrinking tumours, just helping Rob feel better. It has been a very difficult four weeks for us. I have been so, so proud of Rob. He is so tough in his quiet Rob way, he doesn't ever complain, he went without the chemotherapy for far longer than I ever could have. I don't know where he finds the strength to do this, but he does, and every day points out the positives ("well I feel pretty good right this very moment").

The other day he sneaked into the kitchen and emptied the dishwasher when I slipped out to the back yard, just to be helpful, and then was exhausted for the next hour, what a turkey! But that is so Rob; takes a lot to stop him. I'm sure I'll never know everything he's gone through or going through; but it was pretty clear that if Rob felt it was time for him to go back to chemotherapy, he needed to go back.

So, it's not a very uplifting email, but we wanted everyone to know what was happening. Now is when I ask, plead, for everyone to point their own thoughts and prayers towards Rob. He will need all the help and strength he can muster for this next leg of the journey. He needs that web of support now more than ever to hold him up.

Thanks to everyone.

Jen

Thursday 5 August 2010
E-mail from Jen to Helen

Hi Helen,

Forwarding you our latest Rob update, not great news. The beast is back, making its presence known. Chemotherapy tomorrow, Rob is very positive it will work. Bless him for being this way.

I'm on my way up to bed to get him settled and read some Bernie

Siegel. *My current book is "How to Live between Office Visits" to try and help me stay in the present. I skip the chapters on "what to do when children die", not helpful right now.*
Take care,
Jen

Monday 9 August 2010
E-mail from Jen to Helen

It's been a rough few days.
Rob had chemotherapy Friday. His platelets were just above cut off value, much lower than they were before the chemotherapy holiday, which means that's likely his last chemotherapy.
Today and yesterday he had some muddling and confusion, which is apparently likely related to hydromorphone toxicity, so we're facing a possible hospital admission to switch him to methadone. It's hard not to fear what's ahead. It's been rocky.
Talk soon,
Jen

Monday 9 August 2010
E-mail from Helen to Jen

Hi Jen,
Thanks for this latest, I am very sad for/with you about the chemotherapy. It looks like it's come to an end. A big moment and I find tears welling in me with you.
I'm not sure we can ever not fear pain of any kind. All we can do is stay with whatever the 'what is' is; if it is fear, we can cradle it without judging ourselves or fighting it, if it's despair, we cradle that in the same way, breath by breath. It's all we can do and somehow it is all that we need to do, riding the waves as they come, letting them move through us.

So holding it all alongside you, I'm here Jen for you both in what-ever ways I can be present with you.

In breath and prayer, sadness and trust in the great weaving of it all beyond our ability to know or imagine.

Helen

Tuesday 10 August 2010
Rob's Personal Update
"A year and still here …"

Hi everybody. It's Rob. I've never written to you directly before now from my email.

Today marks the one-year anniversary since my diagnosis with meta-static pancreatic cancer. At this point, I share the privilege of being able to write this sentence with only five percent of people with this same diag-nosis after one year. The odds have been against me, but those who know me know that I see every challenge as an opportunity. Jen and I wanted to write a summary of what the year has been. It was a bit startling to do some of the math. Some of the totals (particularly some of the big num-bers) are only conservative estimates, most are accurate.

Our life has changed dramatically over the last year, and we could have only completed this year with all the love and support we have received from friends and family. I never could have imagined the outpouring of support and well wishes that I have received. It has been a humbling ex-perience, and I thank everyone from the bottom of my heart.

I have had many people comment on my strength and courage, but I feel the way I have persevered this year is by living one day at a time, and enjoying each of those days to the fullest. I have created wonderful memories with my family over the past year and had so many important, meaningful conversations I may have never had in the absence of this diagnosis. Not only have I created memories but memories have been cre-ated for me through the events that have unfolded in the past year. For that I am truly thankful.

I have started back to chemotherapy, I may only get a treatment or two before this body of mine starts refusing to cooperate, but for now that's the plan. If I could change the events of the past year to erase this cancer, there's nothing that could stop me. I see the pain that this has caused my family and friends every day, but we have all been on this journey together and the help and support I have received has made the tough items on the list below a lot more bearable. I am positive it's the love and support that has allowed me to still be here today.

Thank you.

So, a summary of my year:

"A year and still here ..."

1 earth shattering terminal diagnosis
3 days in hospital
57 trips to cancer clinic
29 chemotherapy treatments
3 C.T. scans
2 liver biopsies
39 doctor visits
2500 pills/tablets
24 IV lines started successfully (many more unsuccessful attempts)
1 port-a-cath surgery
1100 glucometer readings via lancets
520 insulin injections
150 "other" injections
320 glasses of essiac tea
3 pairs of edema socks
2 edema gloves
22 "Return" airplane tickets purchased by family visiting from England
Over 600 cards of well wishes
1 spectacular "Rob Fazakerley day"
1 wonderful Sisters of St. Jo's award
Uncountable prayers and positive thoughts sent our way
4 trips to Niagara on the Lake

1 family cottage vacation
Many, many tears
Many, many laughs
More love and support from family and friends than we could ever imagine

I'm sure there are lots I've missed, but those were the ones that stood out. Now it's time to shoot for the second year, one day at a time.
Take care, everyone.
Rob

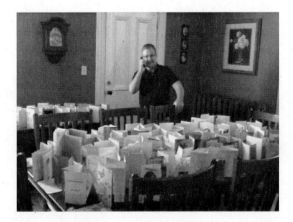

CHAPTER 16

Feeling What He Needs

⌒◯⌒

Thursday 12 August 2010

Jen

I'M SITTING NEXT TO ROB on the couch in our living-room. He's just come downstairs for the morning, hours earlier than usual. He's had a very rough few days and much more pain, and therefore much more pain medication. This morning I can tell something is more wrong. He is confused.

"How are you, Rob?"

"Yes, how am I? I think there is something wrong … Tell me about my doses of drugs … I think we will need to adjust some doses … I think we will need to taper a dose of something … Where are my running shoes? I think I would feel better if I could go for a run. I think I will wear my yellow running shoes. Which drug will we be starting today? I need some breakthrough. I feel nauseous … I think something is wrong. I think I'm a bit loopy. Can you tell me again about my dose of drugs? Something is wrong, Jen. I wouldn't wish this on anyone." And on and on he goes.

Rob is speaking a mile a minute, and he looks afraid. He is asking for pain medicine, nausea medicine, but it doesn't fit with how he seems. I want to go and call Dr. Fryer, but I'm afraid to leave him for even a minute.

I listen to him, sitting right next to him on the couch. In my mind, I start reviewing the past few days and the increased pain medication. I remember from my days of doing clinical work with patients about delirium, and this starts to make sense. For the first time, I hesitate before giving him pain medication. There is a lull in his conversation.

"Rob, I think you may be a little confused this morning. I'm going to stay right here with you. I won't leave you. You will be OK. I'm not going to leave you. Rob, are you having any pain right now?" I ask as calmly as I can, holding his hand. I can feel him calm down as I speak.

"No, I have no pain," he says.

"Rob, can you tell me if you're nauseous at all?" I continue in my most calm voice.

"No, no nausea," he replies quietly.

"OK. Rob, I'm going to call Dr. Fryer and just let her know you're having a rough morning. I'll be right back; I'm just going to get the phone."

This is so worrying, but I realize my instincts were right. I don't think he's having pain — the physical signs aren't there.

As I go to look for the phone, he starts talking again. "So I'm a bit confused, and I'm going to call Dr. Fryer and tell her I want to go for a run. I feel strange. Something's not right. I need breakthrough. I need to get my running shoes. What dose will be the right dose? ... "

I phone the doctor. She is away on holiday. I call Grace and leave a message and then follow up with an e-mail. I hope she is as responsive as she usually is.

Mercifully, Grace calls me back within a few minutes. I sit next to Rob, afraid to leave his side, and talk to Grace. I describe the past several hours and detail the pain medication doses of the past two weeks. I also report on Rob's blood pressure, blood sugar, and a variety of other routine medical details.

Grace listens intently, and then replies, "OK, Jen. I think you're right. It sounds like this confusion is secondary to the increased doses of pain medication he's needed, and no doubt the chemotherapy he's just had has interacted a bit as well. You're doing all the right things.

"You are going to have to rely on what you see and what your gut tells you rather than what Rob says with respect to pain control. He's not going to be able to report accurately. I will connect with some of the doctors here and see if we can strategize what to do next. It sounds like we may need to rotate to another pain medicine. We can bring him into hospital if this becomes unmanageable for you at home."

"No," I respond emphatically, "I'm not having him go to the hospital. I can keep him a lot more calm and comfortable here. It would be horrible for him in the hospital when he's confused like this. I'll figure it out."

Inside, I am emphatic. There is no way he's going into hospital. How would a nurse who doesn't know him possibly know when he does or doesn't need pain medicine?

"OK, Jen. Have you got the kids home with you?" Grace asks.

"Yes." I say. Grace is so on top of this sort of thing. Jack and Haley are both home on summer holidays. I have told them just an hour before that they need to stay in the other room because Rob is having a rough day. I'm not sure how to manage with them and also look after Rob in this state.

"Can they go somewhere else? Could they go to their Dad's? This may get worse before it gets better, and you will need to keep your focus on Rob."

"Yes. Good idea, Grace. I'll arrange that right away," I say, happy for the direction.

"OK, Jen. Hang in there. I'll be in touch with a few of the docs here, and we'll have a plan by lunch. Call if anything changes, and I'll talk to you shortly"

"Thanks, Grace. Bye." What an incredible support she is!

Saturday 14 August 2010

Jen

OVER THE NEXT FEW DAYS, I spend every minute of the day and night fielding the confusion and keeping Rob calm. I can't leave him for even a minute or he becomes worse. It exhausts me, as it goes on day and night. Grace works with doctors at the London Regional Cancer Program to plan medication tweaks, and after a few days things seem to be calming down.

When Dr. Fryer returns from holiday on 14 August, she visits us and we update her. I learn about opioid-induced toxicity and delirium.

"You've weathered quite a storm, Rob," Dr. Fryer comments after examining Rob. The confusion has gone, but not the muscle twitching – another sign of toxicity. She continues, "It's quite amazing that you were able to manage the delirium from home without a hospitalization."

I reply, "I don't know how it ever would have been managed in hospital. It was so difficult to tell what he actually needed, I had to use every bit of gut instinct and intuition I have. I'm so glad we have such a strong connection, because I could feel what he needed, even if it was different from what he was saying. It was really intense."

The doctor explains to us, "Opioid-induced delirium is very difficult to manage in hospital, because we always need to balance the need for pain control with the risk of toxicity. The risk of getting into what we call a 'pain crisis' is very high. Rob is lucky you were able to do it from home and that you never did get into a pain crisis. I think the only reason you could do this from home is that you are very in tune with what Rob's needs are, even when he isn't able to articulate them."

I agree. Despite my exhaustion, I'm deeply grateful we've managed.

Sunday 15 August 2010
Rob Update

Rob had chemotherapy last week. He experienced some challenges afterwards related to the hydromorphone that he takes for pain because during the chemotherapy holiday he had experienced a significant increase in pain and had increased his hydromorphone by a lot. Within a couple days of last week's chemotherapy he experienced some signs of opioid toxicity, which include some involuntary muscle twitching and confusion, no pain though.

Under physician guidance we have now decreased the hydromorphone again, and are trying to find a dose that manages his pain, but does not produce the above side effects. This is a bit of a juggling act, and has been very challenging for Rob and our family.

We went back to the cancer clinic this past Friday to evaluate Rob for a second chemotherapy dose, but were deferred as his platelets were only forty-three, which is the lowest they have ever been. He will continue to be evaluated weekly by the cancer clinic to see if he can have more treat-

ments, but that road may have come to an end. We'll see. The chemotherapy for Rob works very well for pain and symptom management, so
he would certainly like to see if he can get more, but his platelets would
need to recover significantly for that to be the case.

We have received wonderful support these past few weeks as things
have changed on this path we are on. Thank you for all of this. Rob continues to remain positive and optimistic, living one day at a time. His first
year and still here email attracted so many positive responses on his email,
it's been wonderful.

We realized after we wrote it that we got a number wrong in Rob's
list. It was the number of tablets he takes in a year. The list Rob sent said
twenty-five hundred, we missed a zero. It is twenty-five thousand per year.

Take care all,

Jen

Thursday 19 August 2010
Rob Update

After a very difficult couple weeks, Rob is starting to stabilize, and I wanted to tell people. Our palliative care doc did a home visit on Tuesday, and
suggested Rob rotate to a different narcotic from the one that he's been
taking for the past year. So, we're switching to methadone, which many
people will have heard of with respect to heroin addicts, but is also a very
effective narcotic for cancer pain.

This isn't an easy process and one that normally requires a hospital
admission as it requires close supervision and a competent caregiver and
support team. However, breaking new ground as always we are doing this
transition from home, which Rob and I are so relieved about. Neither of us
was looking forward to an admission (I was planning how I would camp
out there without getting in trouble from the hospital administration).

Anyway, great physician, great supportive team, and a 'competent' caregiver; means that we are doing the switch from home and so far so good.
Side effects are clearing; pain management is improving, what more could
we ask?

Well, we asked for 'more platelets' so Rob could have more chemo-therapy and to our surprise we got what we asked for. Rob had some blood work today at Woodstock Hospital (to save us the drive to London) and to our shock and delight his platelets have gone all the way up from forty-three last week to one hundred and nine today, so he's having more chemotherapy tomorrow (Friday). When our palliative care doctor called us to tell us the numbers, she said she had to read them twice because she couldn't believe they had recovered.

Now, I know that several people have specifically prayed for Rob this past week and sent positive energy and whatever else people do. And I also know that there have been some specific requests re: platelets to what-ever higher power people subscribe to. I also know that Rob and I have spent many hours visualizing, praying, hoping, and focusing on giving him strength to fight this and stay here. So, it looks like something or everything has granted Rob the ability to continue his fight, at least for this week.

As I am writing this email, I'm on the couch, writing from my blackber-ry, sitting next to Rob, listening to music on Rob's new ipod through our little stereo. I bought Rob an ipod yesterday as an early Christmas present so he could listen to some of his favourite music and relax when he was lying on the couch (which he's been doing a lot of late). Jessica spent all afternoon loading songs onto the ipod and then as a surprise, and celebra-tion of clearing side effects, new drugs, more chemotherapy and higher platelets, Jessica and I gave it to him at supper tonight.

As I was writing the last paragraph, the song "Let it be" by the Beatles came up. That song has been with me ever since I woke up with it in my head last October, it is my 'meditation' song. It helps me relax in the middle of the night if I find myself looking into a dark future. To me, it car-ries a message of 'leave your troubles to God' and although I've never been terribly religious, this song has helped a lot. So interesting that it pops up when I was writing about the power of prayer and positive thinking. Any-way, I find stuff like this very interesting and spiritual.

(Two songs later was "Lucy in the sky with diamonds", Rob was playing air guitar to the music. So these spiritual moments do come and go as do the little bits of opioid related confusion!)

Anyway, this is a 'good news' email. Rob's in chemotherapy tomorrow, maybe his last, maybe not. Who knows? His willpower is incredible. We've got a treatment plan for new drugs to help with side effects, and so for now, for these next few minutes anyway, things are ok.

Thank you, thank you to every single person who prayed, thought, wished and hoped for Rob these past few days. Rob and I know this has worked some magic and we thank God for that as well as everyone who has sent all of the support and well wishes that we have received.

Thank you everyone.

Please keep the faith.

Jen

Thursday 19 August 2010
E-mail from Helen to Jen

> *Thanks for the update Jen. Amazing synchronicities. Indeed, you are not alone for sure in all this.*
>
> *Have been keeping you all in my prayers and visualizations very much.*
>
> *Helen*

Saturday 21 August 2010
E-mail from Jen to Helen

> *Hi Helen,*
>
> *It's been a tough two weeks. Rob's parents arrive tomorrow for three weeks. I'm glad for Rob that they're coming as he says he's looking forward to the visit. Rob tries to cover up how crappy he feels, which was next to impossible during this past two weeks of opioid induced delirium. Anyway, that seems to be clearing. I'm hoping that this little shot of chemotherapy will help him feel better and be able to enjoy the visit. It will be a busy few weeks.*
>
> *Today is Jack's ninth birthday party, the day after chemotherapy, in the midst of a delirium and a switch to methadone. Life goes on.*

Jack and Haley's dad is coming to help. I wanted the kids to have some memories of an overlap with Rob and Dave (the kids' dad) and to see we're all on the same team for them. It's been an interesting time; tough for the kids to see Rob get worse, but they're still kids.
Take care, Helen.
Jen

Saturday 21 August 2010
E-mail from Helen to Jen

Hey Jen,
Good to hear from you. I am holding you all so closely and am reminded again and again how interconnected we all are, how life supports us in our times of need in these subtle ways. We can't always remember that for ourselves in the tough places, so I hold that for you all. In your shoes it probably feels scary as all get out, overwhelming and bleak.
You are doing amazing Jen, truly. What you are holding with such awareness and the way you are weaving things and following your gut is quite stunning, for example the party and having the two 'worlds' for your children come together briefly. We usually don't see how amazingly well we are doing when we feel inside like we're holding on by our fingernails.
May wind fill your sails and if suddenly you feel becalmed may the sun warm you and give you a moment of rest.
Helen

Sunday 22 August 2010
E-mail from Jen to Helen

Hi, nice to hear from you too.
The party was great. Most importantly the kids seemed to really enjoy all of the love together in the same room. Jack said it was his

best birthday and said what a great birthday he had and he loved Dave and Rob.

My daughter told me she felt so glad when she saw Rob and daddy in the same room and that Rob looked so small (Dave is 6'9").

We just returned from church. Rob said as he was clearing from his delirium on Thursday and had news of being ok for chemotherapy Friday that he wanted to go to church and hear some hymns. First time we've ever entered our little united church here in Norwich, but hymns he got and he said he enjoyed it. Teeny congregation of white haired people and a few forty something, nice minister lady in her mid-fifties, I think, quite contemporary. Funny how our youth calls us in times of stress. Rob grew up going to church every Sunday, all so interesting.

He's clear today cognitively for the first time in two weeks; it's so nice to have him 'back' with me. I think I was preparing myself to say goodbye these past two weeks. So to have him have a little reprieve in his wellbeing and health has sent me firmly into the front seat of the roller coaster and so many emotions. Mostly like I'm not ready and never will be to see him go, no surprise there. It's so raw.

I do feel like I'm holding on by my fingernails and often losing grip. Rob holds me here though. I can keep it all going if I've got him in my mind and hear his voice saying "I'm not going anywhere". I have a feeling that voice will be with me always.

So, that's today.

Take care,

Jen

Monday 23 August 2010

E-mail from Helen to Jen

Hi Jen,

Very touching Jen. The hymns, the party, all so full of life even in the midst of such heartache. Thanks for sharing.

Not sure one is ever 'ready', no such state I don't think, personally.

I do know that whatever happens the experience will have all the simi- lar ingredients that the past year has had: struggle, tears, surprises, heartbreak, totally unexpected gifts, comfort, despair, new discoveries of the meaning of 'hope' and then letting go again and a feeling of life weaving its way through it all, encompassing the pain and whatever words you would put in yourself.

I also trust so deeply that the love is real and that is not mortal. It can't 'disappear' because it's an energy wave, a 'field' of energy as it were, as is Rob. What that means can only be discovered in each moment as it evolves.

Ever joined in your field of energy with my prayers.

Helen

Sunday 29 August 2010
E-mail from Jen to Helen

Hi Helen,

Just wanted to touch base.

We're a week into our visit from Rob's parents. Rob's had some tough days, rotating from hydromorphone to methadone, but has weathered it beautifully as he always does. As his confusion has lifted, I find so many floods of emotions rising to the surface, almost like last chance conversations? Seems odd.

I spoke to Rob's mum last night and tried to convey how deeply I loved Rob, how it has been a privilege to spend this last year caring for him, that I feel that we were meant to come together, that he is an incredible person who has impacted countless people, that we've been so lucky to have all the support from family and friends that we have, and that she raised him well to have him turn out the way he has, and how happy we had been for the last six years.

I find I can't wait to go to bed with Rob at night and have time with just us. This sounds terrible Helen, but I found myself wishing that when he finally takes his last breath, I hope it's there, in our bed, with me by his side. I know it likely won't be, but that's what I found myself thinking last night.

We've been preparing a bit more for that event, doing the 'EDITH' paperwork (expected death in the home), signing "DNR (Do not Resuscitate)" cards, talking to Dr. Fryer about 'what does liver failure look like'. Nothing new that we don't already know (I used to attend meetings about 'EDITH', helped create the paperwork, very bizarre to be using it).

I asked Rob where he was in his 'fight' one night, expecting him to say he was growing weary; he perked right up and started talking about chemotherapy, how he still felt strong, and he wasn't planning on going anywhere for a long time. Ok then.

Fall is around the corner. I'm sitting in my backyard right now. I'm the only one up, looking at the green tufts that were the forget-me-nots. We have loads of brown eyed Susans blooming now that Rob transplanted last spring before he was diagnosed. Makes me sad to think how strong he was, how fast he used to move. It seems like a lifetime ago.

My children have been away for the past three weeks with their dad while things have been rough with Rob and we've done the drug switch. I miss them terribly. Things are so much harder when they're here, more for me to do, but they remind me that there is more than this existence. I can't believe one day I won't be doing this anymore; no more drugs, injections, dosettes, phone calls, chemotherapy.

We'll talk soon
Take care,
Jen

Sunday 29 August 2010
E-mail from Helen to Jen

Hi Jen,

I am quite stunned by how well you're doing all this. 'Well' in the sense of just continuing to fearlessly live it, say the truth, name the 'what is' and grab every moment as you can.

Try asking the universe for your wish, to be beside him at home for the last physical breaths. Put it out there, see it in your mind's eye, and then let it go with the 'whatever's best' kind of inner attitude. But ask. Who knows?

I am also wondering about a mantra like, "Life will support me whatever happens, as it has this past year" as you hit the horror moments of anticipatory grief and when I say 'Life' I mean the vast expansive life force that encompasses death, not life as in the 'opposite' of death but life as in the cycle that pushes the green shoots through the cracks in the concrete.

Mantras work like anchors in the moment, they take how we're feeling, apply a 'truth' that feels true in that moment (i.e. not something that's pie in the sky or beyond our gut's reach) and thus honour how we feel and the reality of hardship but also affirm a perspective that's bigger than the fear or pain.

Always here, Jen. If you'd like a home visit on Tuesday, I could come your way. I'd be happy to meditate with you both and share some time together. Offer's there and I trust you'll honour as always, what feels right for you.

Take care and a big hug to you both.

Helen

Sunday 29 August 2010
E-mail from Jen to Helen

Hi Helen,

I'm so happy you can come. Rob seemed very touched and genuinely surprised that you would come all this way to see him. The first thing he said was "I wonder if Helen might be involved in my funeral?" Rob told his parents you were coming. His mum asked if she could be around for that, Rob said "of course", I said yes.

Thank you Helen, you've meant so much to us over the past year and I know you will continue to be such an important part of our journey. Funeral or not, you've taught me so much about me.

Take care,

Jen

Sunday 29 August 2010
E-mail from Helen to Jen

> Rob's parents can be around for sure, as always, I'll just go with my intuition but I am sensing that a time of meditation together might be valuable.
> See you soon,
> Helen

Monday 30 August 2010
E-mail from Jen to Helen

> Funny how we re-read emails. I re-read the last one I sent you, when I said you'd taught me so much about me, felt fraudulent at three in the morning. I feel like I should have said you have tried to teach me about me, point out things between Rob and I, my 'strength', etc, and ability to cope.
> But I find when you or anyone for that matter, points out how strong I am or how well I'm coping or that I'm doing everything 'right', I don't feel strong or like I'm coping well.
> I feel like I'm neglecting my kids (there's that maternal inadequacy you mentioned, although they are at Canada's Wonderland today with their dad and I guarantee I'm the last thing on their minds), that I panic when I think of Rob at the end of his life here, not calm, not coping. And I feel I'll lose it and never do it without him.
> I have to say it is nice to hear people tell me I'm doing a good job, I just have no yardstick to compare myself to and it doesn't always feel like I'm doing a good anything, just loving Rob. We're so looking forward to seeing you, it has been so long since he's seen you and you always spark such conversations between us long after our sessions.
> My 'needs' are so far at the bottom of the list at the moment, but I know I need you tomorrow, so that's perfect.
> Take care,
> Jen

Monday 30 August 2010
E-mail from Helen to Jen

Hi Jen,

That's why I keep telling you that you ARE doing a good job and mirroring what I see because I actually DO have a 'yardstick' in a way!

I see many people in not dissimilar situations and I see the full array of coping styles and mechanisms people have to deal with pain, at the core, no negative judgment, but all 'coping skills' are not created equal. So just take it in blind faith that you ARE doing amazingly well. And there's no wool being pulled, at least not on my eyes.

You've never tried to be more than you are as a way of coping. And, guaranteed, without him physically present, after his passing over, you WILL lose it, you WILL feel like you've gone out of your mind, you WILL feel like everything is utterly meaningless.

Expect it then you don't have to try to do anything to prevent that experience. Just expect the full gamut of human despair and do what you've done through this whole journey, be with it, stay with it, live into it instead of away from it and even that despair will be a river that takes you somewhere different, if you allow it to.

And you cannot be everywhere at all times and be what you need to be for everyone. Be the mother you are, a mother living heartbreak. Show them that you are doing what you need to do for yourself, for Rob, which you are. They'll survive you not being there for them in all the ways you think you should be. They know they are loved. Your parents, their grandparents are holding them well. That's all that really is needed.

And just in case you try to remember anything I've said, don't! Grief will work its way in and through you and you will come out different. You as you know yourself and your life as you've known it will die with Rob. That is a fact. And you will rebirth a new life. You don't want to, it's the last thing that you want to have to do, but it will happen. A new life will work its way into you and through you.

You can't will it to happen or therapize it into being. But grief lived into takes you into a new life, green shoots pushing through concrete, spring following winter. That much I do trust and believe with my heart and soul.

And Rob will be there in ways you can't even imagine, whether you feel him or not. He will be. That too I trust.

See you tomorrow at your house. Looking forward to it.

Helen

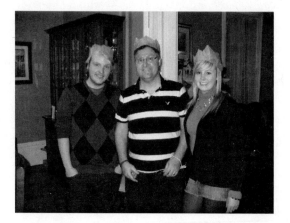

CHAPTER 17

The Family Circle

∞

Tuesday 31 August 2010
Fifth Spiritual Care Session

Helen

I AM DRIVING TO Jen and Rob's home. It is not on work time, since my scope does not reach to home visits on part-time hours, but, once again, my gut has guided me to this 'stretch' decision. They cannot come to the clinic — Rob's precious energy is far too low now. And the inner truth is I also need to see him one more time. I need to say my own goodbye.

Rob's parents, Brian and Mildred, are there too, English people from near my parent's roots in the north. I wonder what this visit will be like. Rob and Jen and I have shared a very sacred and in many ways invisible journey, involving some rather unusual conversations and meditations. How will I integrate his folks into this time together? Jen has suggested we might have time just the three of us, but who knows? — these visits with family have a tendency to unfold in unanticipated ways.

I drive up to their home. It resonates with my own passion for old, English-style houses and stirs my own homeland longing. I can see why Rob would have fallen in love with it. It is quintessentially the English manor house. I had no idea they lived in such a home. They'd described it, but it is much larger than I'd imagined and totally gorgeous. Old yellow brick with red shutters, a funny, turret-style front porch that seems oddly incongruent with the rest.

Two small dogs out on a leash greet me with their barks. I get out of the car and pause, taking in the feeling of the place. It's very peaceful, tranquil even. I feel grounded and at home and can somehow feel the stories all around me. This is a place where other people have lived and died. Jen and Rob's story is weaving into its history.

I take a deep breath with a prayer, "May this be all that it needs to be; may I be guided and allow whatever needs to happen to flow through our time together." I have a sense that we will meditate together, including Brian and Mildred. This is for them too, my intuition is suggesting.

I go to the door, and Jen is there to greet me. We hug. Different context, in her home. She is welcoming me now as I've welcomed them into my office space for our sessions. A turning is beginning.

I enter and see a lovely kitchen, bright and airy. Mildred comes from another room, and I meet her. Jen takes me through into the living-room, and there on the large sectional couch sits a man. I think that it's Rob's Dad, but I reach out my hand and realize, as he takes it, that it's Rob. My goodness, how much he has changed! His swelling with the oedema is so much more, and he clearly is not going to waste energy to stand. I reach over to hug him warmly.

"Hi, Rob, it's so good to see you."

He smiles, and our eyes meet; again that steady gaze of his meets mine. I can see he knows that I didn't quite recognize him at first, but he is forgiving, I see that gratefully.

We all sit down, his parents next to Jen on the couch. I sit next to Rob's feet, which he has stretched out across the corner seat, leaving space at his feet. I want to be close to him and looking at him as I take him in.

"How are you doing, Rob?" I ask, opening the way for conversation.

"Oh, all right. It's nice to have my Mum and Dad here with us." He looks over at them.

"Yes, from my homeland!" I affirm warmly. "My parents are from Manchester and Chapel-en-le-Frith in Derbyshire." His parents grab onto this connection, and we chat about England and our common roots. Light streams in through the living-room windows. I feel, again, a sense of warm light, as I always have with Jen and Rob in my office. I'm not sure it's just the sun I'm noticing.

Rob shares stories about the cottage and how good it was for them to go. How things have changed "a bit" since then and the chemotherapy holiday extended, but now he's trying some cycles again to keep things at bay some more. They're hoping very much it will.

Ben and Jessica come into the room — I have not met her before. I am not sure how Rob and Jen and I can meditate with his parents and children present. I feel a sense of peace, however, and trust that the right moment will appear.

Jen is telling me, "There's been a lot of changes, Helen, in the past few weeks since the cottage. The opioid-induced delirium was quite the roller coaster, but we managed to switch him over to another pain medication at home, which is almost unheard of. He's much better with the pain now, and the delirium has gone. Thank goodness. Rob was really out of it!"

She shares with us some of the funny things he had said in his delirium, and we laugh. Even delirious, he is charming and gentle.

"And how are you doing this visit?" I ask his parents. I wonder what their son's dying must be like for them, with home and friends three thousand miles away. Mildred tells us how glad they are to be here, that they hoped to see Rob again after their previous trips but weren't sure. I feel the same towards my ageing parents whenever I visit them in England.

I ask Jessica how she is and comment on my admiration for her sustaining university through all this. The moment has come. A slight shift in the light. A subtle current in the room's energy brings the talking to a natural pause.

"I wonder if you'd like to share a time of meditation together." I want them all to feel welcome, if they wish to participate.

Jen and Rob nod very affirmatively, as does everyone else. The unanimous consent surprises and heartens me. The group meditation may nourish them in meaningful ways.

"So let's just close our eyes and gently become aware of our breath and feeling our feet on this ground beneath us. Feel the solidness of the earth below that is supporting us even in the many waves of feelings that come and go, that ground is always there," I begin, as I always do, breath and earth, the two anchors for any storm.

I guide them through a very simple breath-awareness exercise and imagining drawing the breath through the feet. It short-circuits the mind chatter and usually becomes a very grounding and centring experience.

I can feel the energy in the room concentrating. Everyone is present, very present. Again, the sense of light, even though I have closed my eyes, and the centre of it is coming from Rob. I notice this with curiosity. I wonder how close he is to dying and if it's closer than we have been thinking. He feels like a husk that is breaking open with its essence beginning to pour out.

"And as we notice our breath, let's bring into our awareness all the trees that are breathing with us right now, sharing their oxygen, sustaining us and we them. Think of all the oceans that are circulating the water that gives us life and endlessly change from one state to another yet always remaining the same. Just spend a moment considering the web of life that in this moment is living and breathing with us, in which we are all intimately interconnected. One breath, one web."

It feels as if we have become one breath in the room. A shared breath, filling and emptying. A density of energy and a warm yellow radiance very subtly stream between us all.

"And now let's bring our awareness to one another in the room, keeping our eyes closed. Feel into the presence of one another, notice what you feel as you imagine one another around you, notice what comes to your mind's eye. We are all energy forms, interconnected, distinct, yet all part of the same web of life."

This is a slightly more challenging step, but my intuition is nudging me there. Jen and Rob have embraced this deeply. It may provide some comfort for the others if they can touch into that experience of the 'other' as deeply interconnected.

"And now imagine that we are all connected in a circle, breathing together, breathing one breath, because in a way, we are. This connection is the very heart of life. Death might change the form, but it can't change the interconnectedness that we are.

"And a way you can be with Rob on the heartline, even from three thousand miles away, is to focus on him, in your mind's eye, and send your prayers, your heart energy, to him with a phrase such as, 'I am with you,' imagining an energetic thread connecting your heart to his and breathing all your love and care through it to him. You breathe in with his pain or suffering, and you breathe out your prayer for what he needs in that moment. This is an ancient practice, and he will feel it. It's very real." A thread offered. Nothing more.

We sit in silence for a few moments, breathing in the interconnected circle that we've become for a few brief moments. The warmth and light are inwardly palpable, I can feel they're all fully engaging.

"Now, gently bring your awareness back to your body in the room, to yourself. Notice how you feel. Gently, open your eyes and come back to the room when you're ready."

I pause to give everyone time to adjust to having their eyes open and digest the experience a bit.

"What did you notice? If you'd like to share, feel free; if not, that's fine too."

Jen responds right away, "That was incredible, as always, Helen. I felt like I could sense everybody's energy in the room, and it was wonderful to have the feeling of everyone's energy harnessed, giving messages to Rob." Her eyes are bright and alive.

Rob's are too, as he adds, "I felt very peaceful. I could feel everyone in the room." I have no doubt he felt a great deal.

His mother adds: "That was very relaxing," she begins, with a touch of amazement in her voice. "And I could see almost a yellow light coming into the room."

This really touches me. I wasn't the only one inwardly 'seeing' a yellow light. This was new for them. I'm so glad they stayed.

I don't belabour the sharing, as I don't want Ben and Jessica to feel they have to speak. I continue, "This is a way you can stay very connected to each other even from England. It's a powerful practice called tonglen, and I do believe, personally, that it strengthens our connection so that, even after we die, we can stay present to one another across that threshold. That's something Jen, Rob, and I have been exploring and sharing about in our journey together."

I really hope that it may give Rob's parents some comfort after they leave. It's time for me to go. I can feel the 'ending' of our time together, as if the door has opened and the energy is leaving the room.

I stand up to say my goodbyes. I look at Rob and hug him; I look at him, knowing I may not see him again. This is my goodbye. But I don't make it obvious or formal. That would be way too intrusive.

I have said many goodbyes like this in my time as a chaplain. Endings have become as familiar as beginnings, but they don't become any easier. I will feel a significant loss when Rob dies. He's an incredible man and has embodied something I had never met in someone facing death for such a long period: absolute and utterly authentic equanimity. He has been a profound teacher. Inwardly, I give Rob a deep, deep bow, and I feel the tears pricking my eyes.

"Goodbye, Rob." I see his eyes holding mine; he knows what I'm saying. "I carry you deeply in my heart and will in the days ahead." He nods. He knows.

Jen and I hug. What a brave woman. She has walked this knife edge with such dignity, courage, and honesty. I know in this moment that our journey will not end with Rob's death. This experience has etched deep into both of our lives, and the arc of this relationship we've forged, the three of us, will not end with his death.

Somehow, my gut tells me, we will journey together through the treacherous path of grief, and I will continue to be a Sherpa with her in that wilderness too. I sense the call to keep holding the candle for Jen in the dark, dark hours ahead, trusting, when she may not be able to, that life will show up for her, somehow, some way, and that Rob will find a way too to comfort her. I give this awareness silently, inwardly to Rob as my parting gift.

I hug Brian and Mildred, Ben and Jessica, and leave their family circle. I've done what I came to offer. Their circle needs to close now around Rob and Jen. The journey ahead is a sacred one.

Jen accompanies me to the back door and offers to show me their garden. We walk around to the back. She looks, with a weighty sadness, at their beautiful flagstone patio and pond. She points to it: "We built that together. Rob loved to do things around this house and garden. We both did. We spent a weekend building that when the kids weren't here. We spent so much of our kid-free time together at Home Depot. We used to joke and say we should get a franchise or shares!"

I take in the garden; it's very beautiful, English style, and feels as old as the hills, as most gardens back home do. I can feel Rob has a resonance similar to mine with the old hills and moors of northern England where he lived and my roots are. Something ancient, wild, and beautiful about it, his transplant into a rural township in Ontario. I love it immediately.

"He won't be here to get it ready in the spring," Jen adds, again that sadness running through her words like an underground river. "He always took care of the pond pump and got it going. He loved working outside in the garden. He loves our house."

Again, the sense of this home's having its own journey, soul life, calling them here to bring it back to life, and with that the aching awareness of the challenges ahead for Jen. So much that one loses in losing a partner. She's facing the life of the single mother and householder as well, and that is no easy task.

"It's been such a roller coaster, the last month," Jen continues, "with the delirium, then clearing it, and all the medication changes. I know we don't have very long," she pauses, and I feel the ache she's feeling almost palpably in my own chest. "You must see that," she adds.

I nod quietly. I do.

Jen pauses and then continues, "I've never really talked to you about the intimate part of our relationship, but I just have to tell you this, it is so strange. Even with his health really starting to fail and the delirium and all the medication changes over the past several weeks, something's happened with Rob physically that we've been able to enjoy some intimacy again. It's been amazing and so weird. It has certainly heightened the highs and lows of the past few weeks, and it's made me realize, even more, how terribly I'm going to miss him."

This strikes me powerfully. "Well, that's wonderful, Jen. He's finding his way to you even in the midst of all that is happening physically."

I also sense that this means it will not be long before he dies. I see in my mind's eye the last burst of colour before the flowers go to seed in late summer, returning to the soil. This feels like a last burst of life energy before his body fails.

But another thought comes to me unbidden. I wonder whether this is somehow alchemizing his 'energy body' in quantum metabolic and energetic levels in his connection with Jen. Whether, somehow, he is intuitively, beyond any cognitive awareness, strengthening their shared field of energy so that they will find each other through their connection on the heartline after his death. Nothing that we'll ever know for sure, but in the quantum realm, of which we know so little, it is possible.

We say goodbye with a hug. My sense is that the next time I see Jen she will be alone, without Rob. I offer a silent prayer of thanks for the undercurrent that guided, sustained our time together. And I say a prayer, a hope against hope, that Rob will find his way to Jen, somehow, when his body has returned to the earth.

Tuesday 31 August 2010
E-mail from Jen to Grace

> *Here is where I am so glad you are a female, and Dr. Fryer is a female, because I certainly wouldn't be sharing this kind of info otherwise.*
>
> *Amidst the methadone switch, the in-laws visiting, the nausea and the breakthrough pain, Rob has enjoyed resumption in sexual function for the time being. Creativity abounds! I'm sure you can imagine Grace how this helps to amplify the peaks and valleys of the past couple weeks from my perspective, Rob's too I'm sure. The first instance was at the tail end of his confusion with some interesting disinhibited conversation about how he thought my boobs had shrunk!*
>
> *Forgive me, but who else am I going to tell this stuff?*
>
> *Anyway, a little gift during all these days of picking funeral hymns.*
>
> *And clearly, with present company in house, this will not be a living room conversation for today, but you already knew that.*
> *Jen*

Wednesday 1 September 2010
E-mail from Jen to Grace

> *We're here at the cancer clinic as I write this. Saw the oncologist. He examined Rob's belly, asked if Rob was still interested in continuing in "this hassle", (chemotherapy) Rob said, "absolutely."*
>
> *He had not heard about Rob's delirium, etc., seemed surprised, and wanted to know how Dr. Fryer had done the methadone switch at home.*
>
> *Yesterday was good, Rob was happy to have done the Expected Death in the Home (E.D.I.T.H.) paperwork. You were great as always.*
>
> *Take care,*
> *Jen*

Wednesday 1 September 2010
E-mail from Grace to Jen

> *Hi Jen,*
>
> *Sorry to miss you. Been kind of a nutsy day.*
>
> *I spoke with the oncologist. He filled me in. And a 'custom chemotherapy' schedule sounds like a good idea. Hopefully this will satisfy Rob's platelet production centre.*
>
> *Sorry that he didn't have an update regarding the Methadone before your visit. He was impressed!*
>
> *Hope your afternoon with Helen went well. Did she get to meet Rob's parents?*
>
> *Hopefully, these next couple weeks provides some ease in your day to day being. You could use that I think!*
>
> *Be in touch!*
> *Grace*

Wednesday 1 September 2010
E-mail from Jen to Grace

Hi Grace,

No worries about the oncologist not knowing about the metha-done. I had told the nurse and she had written it down and clearly he didn't have time to read that note either. Glad to hear he was impressed, we aim to please you know!

Helen was wonderful, she met Rob's parents and Ben and Jessica, and led us in a group meditation session of 'tonglen' at the end of her session, which was powerful and impressive. Rob was whipped by the end of yesterday, but so pleased with how the day went. I was so touched, humbled, and moved that she came on her own time, which is just how I feel when you answer your cell phone or email me back on your weekends or holidays or our palliative doctor. We are so lucky to have you all.

So, I hope for a wee break of calm as well. And yes I could really use it.

Take care,

Jen

Wednesday 1 September 2010
E-mail from Grace to Jen

So glad you had a good session with Helen. I hope all found it as meaningful. I am quite certain they too would have been grate-ful for her presence. And never worry, we're here for you. For Rob, the kids, everyone! We're all here to do right by you! And a great privilege to be sure.

Talk again,

Grace

Thursday 2 September 2010
E-mail from Jen to Grace

> *Hi Grace,*
> *I was telling my mum about the oncologist appointment yesterday as she was here with the kids, yesterday. I was telling her how, after telling him all about the delirium and drug changes, I said (quoting you) "so I think we've been through quite a storm, but got through it."*
> *He looked down, and while writing something said "oh yes, and many more big waves to come." I felt quite annoyed and perhaps, defensive. A reassuring sentence about a few 'better days' to come (temporarily of course) would be most welcome for these weary caregiver types. I think this type of moment is a 'side-effect' of the system. There is so little time to spend with us and stacks more people in the waiting room, all of whom are dying; and perhaps he was intending it to be comforting, who knows. Hope is such a tricky thing to navigate in these oncology conversations.*
> *Today Jessica gets moved back to university. Well, her stuff anyway. I don't think she herself is leaving until Sunday. A lot of emotion for her and Rob as another year starts with a dark unknown on the horizon. I know she finds this hard to see him like this.*
> *Talk soon Grace,*
> *Jen*

Friday 3 September 2010
Rob Update

Rob has weathered a very tough storm these past few weeks, but is feeling a bit better these past few days. We had Rob's monthly oncologist appointment Wednesday. Unfortunately Rob's platelets were once again too low to proceed with chemotherapy for today. Rob's oncologist has invented a custom schedule to try and squeeze out a few more treatments. We are once again reminded of our unique situation, as most patients with pancreatic cancer never run into this problem more than a year post diagnosis. I suppose we're keeping the oncologist on his toes!

Seeing Rob so ill over the past month has catapulted our family once again into some very difficult discussions and decisions about what is to come. It has always been our style as a couple to plan things in advance, prepare for what is to come, and then ride whatever wave comes, knowing we can accomplish almost anything together. So, we have initiated many discussions not because things are imminent, but because we want to be ready, and Rob wants to be involved. As always, these impossibly difficult conversations are smoothed by the skillful, caring words of those who have guided and helped us on this journey.

Our nurse practitioner, Grace managed to navigate through "expected death in the home" paperwork with such "grace" it was almost painless and the visit ended with smiles all around. When asked by us, Dr. Fryer has been reassuring about end stage disease, and pain and symptom management at that time, which is obviously a worry to all of us. So her words have helped ease much fear. Our spiritual care person Helen made a special trip to our home to see Rob and also spent time with his parents and Ben and Jessica. It was an incredible experience.

We are incredibly blessed to have such amazing support from our families, our friends and our health care team, and that has become very apparent in the past four weeks. We have been the recipients of many, many home cooked meals, gift cards for food and pharmacy supplies, and cards and e-mails of support and well wishes.

We are part way through enjoying another visit from Rob's parents, which has been lovely for all of us, especially Rob of course. My garden has never looked as good thanks to the skilled hands of Rob's English parents. Each visit from them is a gift for Rob, as he has the opportunity to sit and reminisce about his childhood and years gone by. My parents have been helping with many day to day comings and goings of our busy house, including moving Jessica back to university, helping with childcare, back to school shopping, laundry, etc, etc. I couldn't do this without them.

We are hoping and praying for a peaceful little patch before the next 'storm' and a few platelets to boot to give Rob the strength to accept the chemotherapy to keep him going. We know we will go through many storms in the coming weeks and months, but I believe that Rob's courage, resilience, and unshakable will power to stay with his family have helped him overcome this last difficult patch. One that I'm sure many people would have taken as a 'final call' and given up, but he didn't. It is these qualities, in combination with all the support we receive that keeps Rob with us, and in his words "I've got lots of living left to do, I'm not going anywhere".

I think that's all. Thank you everyone for all the support, it has been humbling, uplifting, and so very helpful.

Jen

Saturday 4 September 2010
E-mail from Helen to Jen

Beautiful description of your experience Jen. Amazing really. Again, I just feel awe as one does in front of a mystery, gratitude at how you're doing it, who knows, but you are. And remember, all of us around you that you speak of so highly (and thank you for the esteem, it's humbling) are merely reflecting you and Rob back to you, truly.

The visit was very special indeed. I am blessed as much as you are. Big hugs to you both. Holding you very closely in my heart.
Helen

Saturday 4 September 2010
E-mail from Jen to Helen

Well if ever the heartline works it is now. Having a tough morning here with Rob, and I'm sitting in the rocking chair in our room next to the bed as he rests. I have my blackberry with me. I grabbed it out of the kitchen on my last dash downstairs to see if you had written back. I felt like I needed a dose of Helen or Grace. I was just re-reading the e-mail update I sent you yesterday and then your message came in, amazing communication device. (The heartline, not my blackberry).

I've been thinking a lot of your visit and all that you said. The meditation; it was such a powerful few minutes. Funny, I could sense everyone with their own interesting postures and auras.

Rob found it very powerful.

Must go, he's rousing.

Take care,

Jen

Saturday 4 September 2010

E-mail from Helen to Jen

So glad.

Will stay close to Rob on the heartline! It works better than blackberrys.

So, there is a huge circle around you and Rob visible and invisible, you are part of a web that you probably can't even imagine yet but it's showing itself to you both bit by bit and each 'opening' readies you for the next one. I am very convinced Rob is 'training' for something beyond anything we can see or know. As are you, and together you have been creating something that will evolve even when he's on the 'other side of the veil'.

I remember sharing early on about I read a book about a couple who experienced this. He died, he was much older and she realized he was in a sphere that he and her were still deeply connected and he was still partnering with her in this realm 'from the other side', a symbiotic evolving.

This is not a platitude to placate. As always our human bodied self needs to feel the heartache and pain and grief, and you will, and it must be honoured. But, something more evolves through the portal of grief, if we stay open and in it until.

Helen

Saturday 4 September 2010
E-mail from Jen to Helen

It's been a long day. I feel very weary. Rob didn't get out of bed until noon, was confused and lots of pain this morning. Then had a fine afternoon, but exhausted after dinner, and has been in bed since eight. I hadn't even put the little kids to bed by then, so put him to bed first, then the kids, then I had a bath, and I'm just waiting until ten thirty when I can wake him up for his last dose of methadone, then bed.

I do sometimes sense the 'web' we've weaved. I sense it in the hour after I send out my Rob updates. Maybe it's a ripple of energy coming our way as people open the e-mails. I know it's far reaching.

The funny thing is that I just heard from a friend that the e-mails are talked about, e-mailed about, met about during coffee breaks and lunch at Parkwood Hospital, that Rob and I and our journey are the topics of endless conversations, that the e-mails help everyone prioritize their lives, that they make people feel connected and included. And that people talk about how strong I am, and what an incredible person Rob is.

Yet I hear very little from anyone after I send them out into the ether. I never even know when they're distributed. As I send it to one person, and she forwards them on to the group it is the strangest experience, but I can feel it somehow.

I will say goodnight.
Talk soon, heartline or otherwise,
Jen

Saturday 4 September 2010
E-mail from Helen to Jen

You are sensing in a deep way Jen. Just want to affirm that. I trust it deeply. You have no idea how your journey is creating a 'dreaming' or 'net weaving' amongst people and the earth far and wide. But it is.

How do I know? Because of the strength of the heartline I experience with you and Rob. This is not 'typical' or a given with everyone. So whatever is being 'dreamed' in and through us by the great web of life, I've no idea but something is.

Love your updates, thank you.

Helen

Stay with Every Feeling

∞

Tuesday 7 September 2010
E-mail from Jen to Grace

> *Hi Grace,*
> *I understand Dr. Fryer has e-mailed you about Rob's latest large boulder, pulmonary embolisms.*
> *Anyway, just wanted to keep you in the loop, and wanted you to keep me in the loop. Rob's parents scheduled to leave Friday so lots of anxiety around this latest as you can imagine.*
> *Jen*

Friday 10 September 2010
E-mail from Jen to Grace

> *Hi Grace,*
> *The house is quiet. My kids have gone to their dad's for the weekend, Jessica's settled into school, Rob's parents are waiting to board their plane in Toronto and at the moment Rob's sleeping after a long week.*
> *The chemotherapy nurses' faces said it all today. Not one of them knew what to say when Rob said he had a bunch of pulmonary em-*

boli. They just all looked horrified. The visiting nurse the same. It's hard to do the day to day, live for the moment thing when the near future appears to be so clearly painted on everyone's face.

Yet, we do. We have to. But this has certainly hung a cloud above us and it's the first tears I've seen Rob shed since last Christmas.

Take care,

Jen

Saturday 11 September 2010
E-mail from Jen to Helen

Hi Helen,

I was thinking a lot about you yesterday. We were at the London Regional Cancer Program, the mood in chemotherapy was so different as Rob's chart had a requisition on the front from Grace for an ECG (Electrocardiograph) to look at his heart function in lieu of the clots in his lungs. 'Multiple pulmonary emboli' certainly took the spring out of the chemotherapy nurses' step.

Rob looked awful. His colour is very purply red in his face. He's short of breath. This is the face of the end nearing. I know it. He knows it. They definitely knew it. He's still Rob of course. Said goodbye to his parents yesterday, he said as we were driving to chemotherapy "I'm confident we'll see them again, I feel like I still have time."

All that being said, a tough day. I had a thought last night at about midnight, as his breathing was so labored beside me, and it was just us in the house (kids at their dad's, Ben at Justin's, Jessica at university), that he may choose a time like this to slip away when it was just us alone.

However, he was still very much alive first thing this morning wanting his breakfast, though now a bit muddled. It's going to be a tough next few days/weeks.

I have turned away all offers of visitors today, just need time together. Amazing how little of that we've had.

Last night after I put Rob to bed I had an hour and a half to 'wait' until it was time for his methadone. I came downstairs and found a book a friend, who recently lost her dad, had sent, "On Grief and Grieving" by Elisabeth Kubler-Ross. I had a bath and read about her famous 'stages', it was really powerful. It was her last book before she died.

I've never read anything by her and when the friend gave me the book (the week before we left for the cottage) I was horrified, because he wasn't dead yet and at that point still looked far from it. But, went rummaging to find it last night and did. I found myself feeling so afraid of the stages (I've only read the introduction about anticipatory grief and the first chapter on 'the stages'), just wondering how I will ever get through it, how my children will. How will I parent my kids and keep a house running and grieve? And I suppose also go to work to support myself?

I realized last night reading this, the hole that will be created in my life will not only be from losing Rob, but also losing 'looking after Rob', which has taken increasingly more and more of my waking and 'should be' sleeping days and nights. It's terrifying. And so, so sad.

I just disassembled the kids' bunk beds last week. They had been in Haley's room and I split them up once again to provide a bed for Jessica's room to replace the one she took to university. Brought back many memories of the time on my own, after I left my first marriage and bought those bunk beds. It was shortly after that when I met Rob, again, and I always described it feeling like he had a fish hook through my chest, and was pulling me out of dark water towards the light. I walked down the 'aisle' (in our living room) to "angel" by Sarah McLachlan, "pulled from the wreckage" always struck a chord.

So much harder to lose him just six years later.

I've never loved anyone like this, in this way.

Take care. Thanks for e-mailing.

Jen

Saturday 11 September 2010
E-mail from Helen to Jen

Hi Jen,

As you think about the grief ahead remember that your mind can only imagine the loneliness as a black hole. Your mind cannot know that when you are standing keening in your kitchen a bird will come and feed near your window and you'll suddenly feel comforted by something greater than the grief.

It cannot know that when you are breathing one breath at a time with a knife in your heart, a friend will call and you will receive just enough comfort to take you to the next day.

It cannot know that when March and April feel like utter despair and the hole opens up and swallows you, that in that darkness a subtle illumination begins to be noticed and you realize that the abyss is in fact also the fount of life from which everything flows, and you would have missed that illumination, the fertility of the dark pain, had you had any energy to run away from it and band aid it with all the things you used to in the lesser griefs.

Your grief will shape you, mould you, take you into a descent right to the belly of life and there, you may discover that it is in fact a womb of rebirth. There is no way out, only through. It's the eye of the needle.

The only task; stay with every feeling, stay with every breath, reach for comfort when you need it, don't try to do it alone. Keen much and often as the waves hit, sleep lots, keep eating, watch for the green shoots and then watch for survivor's guilt as you begin to have moments of feeling alive again and know that life encompasses you, encompasses death, encompasses Rob and this will be the grand canyon of your life, etched by the grief into something incredible and beautiful that people say, "how come you're so ... (fill in the blank)?"

Your grief will take you places you cannot even imagine right now but what your imagination will always miss in the reaching forward into the future and wondering about it is the incredible forces of life that show up right inside the heart of darkness.

Your emotional honesty is such an incredible strength you have Jen. It's a healing gift.

And a really tough goodbye for his parents, I'm sure.

Your life story is one hallmarked by walking the tough road with dignity and courage; you keep showing up despite the pain and grief. You will find that strength in you on the road ahead which right now only looks like a horror from this side of it. And if life can provide you with Rob to draw you into living again, it can and will do that again in sundry ways again. It will never be what it was with Rob but it won't be the end of your story about your relationship with life giving you what you need.

And without wanting to jump ahead but also aware that it's closer now than it was, I'd be happy to offer to be involved in Rob's funeral by writing something of my journey with you both and reading it, perhaps that could be the reflection part of the service, if you like. I certainly want to be there, for my own sake as well as yours. I wonder if the minister from the church would be willing to officiate?

Right there alongside you both. I can feel Rob's inner strength so deeply when I 'tune in' to him. His body is a dark colour but his inner self, I guess the buddhists would call it his 'energy body' seems very strong and changes colours, like a 'rainbow body' that I've read about in stories of lamas (masters/gurus).

Into the night with prayers.

Helen

Saturday 11 September 2010
Rob Update

A brief update for circulation. Some people on this list have received this information and some haven't. So thought I should update to dispel any inaccurate information.

Rob had some shortness of breath on Monday (Labour Day), and after a battery of tests in Woodstock on Tuesday the 7th, he has been found to have multiple small pulmonary embolisms. He's been started on daily fragmin (blood thinner) injections (by me) to hopefully prevent more clots and stabilize the existing ones. He did have chemotherapy yesterday, a reduced dose. His platelets just squeaked above where they needed to be at eighty one, so chemotherapy proceeded.

Our team of palliative care doctor, nurse practitioner and oncologist are working together to determine how to balance the low platelets with the risk of treating clots with blood thinners, and the risk of bleeding (internally or otherwise) while being on blood thinners. So there is much tweaking of doses, chemotherapy and blood thinners, and much balancing of risks/benefits.

Clots throughout the body are a risk associated with cancer. So this is not unexpected and not uncommon, but is very, very scary. Rob is hopeful that the treatment will stabilize things with his breathing etc., and hopeful that the chemotherapy will help with pain etc. I think that's all for now.

Talk soon,

Jen

Sunday 12 September 2010
E-mail from Jen to Helen

It would mean so much if you could write and read something when the time comes. I was going to call the minister after her church service and see if she would come out to discuss funeral planning.

I certainly recognize the 'stages' from the last year. I'm in a new one now, maybe resignation/acceptance. I know things are coming to a close and I feel the need to get things in order so I can focus on being with Rob. Between listening to breaths and aching in my heart, I make lists of songs, write obituaries, headstones, phone calls; all in my head. I think I do that to force my right brain to take over and give the left side a break, it happens literally in seconds; the flip back and forth, between his breaths. I wonder if others do that.

Take care, Helen,

Jen

Monday 13 September 2010
Visit with Grace

Jen

ROB HAS PULMONARY emboli, diagnosed Tuesday 7 September, and has been on anti-coagulants. I am wondering if his continuing shortness of breath means he needs oxygen. I asked Dr. Fryer, and she suggested he come into Woodstock Hospital to have an O_2 sat. (oxygen saturation) test. I wondered if Grace had a portable machine, and the good news was that she did. She arrives today with it in hand.

"His O_2 sats are fine at rest, but I want to see them when he's challenged." Grace says. "I think this is a dramatic change, and these stairs are going to be a big problem for him. And it's going to be increasingly challenging."

We get Rob upstairs, and his oxygen saturations are fine, but the effort has clearly exhausted him.

I look at Grace's face and watch her watching him, ever reading the silent signals. I tuck him into bed. "Can you hang on when you get downstairs, Grace?" I ask her. I settle Rob and go down to join her. It's time for a conversation.

"How is this going to play out, Grace?"

"What do you mean?" she asks. I sense she knows I am asking about prognosis and timelines, but she wants to be sure.

"I need to know what the trajectory is, based on what you've seen today." I brace myself: Grace always answers our questions honestly, when we're ready to ask them.

"We always say the same thing in palliative care," she says, measuring her words. "It's always weeks to months, days to weeks, or hours to days. What I saw today is a dramatic change, but I don't think we're at hours to days, yet." She is being more careful in how she speaks than I've ever seen before.

The word 'hours' shocks me. Even though it's "not yet," that phrase means it's on the horizon. I realize that in the spaces between the words, in the undercurrent, she is telling me to ready myself for Rob's end of life. It takes about a minute for me to turn my face towards it. I realize that I'm there.

We're there.

I instinctively know in that moment that Rob is there. The horizon that has been moving away from us in the form of 'more time,' which has filled these past months, our present moment, and our days together, is now here.

His dying is beginning.

"So what's this going to look like then, Grace?" I ask, pulling on my left brain to rescue me from the waiting deluge that could break through and never end.

Grace pulls a book out of her bag. "I know we tend to treat you, Jen, like you're a nurse, but I also try to remember that you're not, and especially now. In this book there are some things that may be helpful for you to know about."

I take the book. Grace's timing, as ever, perfect. This is not a volume I could have laid hands or eyes on even a couple of weeks ago: *A Caregiver's Guide: A Handbook about End-of-Life Care*. I take a deep breath and ask her, "What am I to expect?" I need her to guide me through this, as well as a book. I need her to tell me in her reassuring voice.

"We've seen a very steep decline in the last few days, and if this decline continues as it is, you'll see that he has even less energy than now. He'll take to his bed, he'll lose interest in all things around him, he'll lose interest in food and drink, he'll become more dependent on you and the nurse for everything, and that's what will happen. The next two weeks will be very telling."

I remember the conversation six months earlier that Rob had initiated. How he was preparing me for this moment. Now, it's me asking the question, and we're here. Grace's body language is telling me more than the words, we're here.

"He'll get to the point of not being able to get up and down stairs, and you'll either have to get a bed downstairs or move him to hospice," Grace adds.

We're not moving him to hospice. This I know. I say emphatically, "Rob has always been very clear he wants to die at home, and so I want to do everything we can to keep him at home."

Grace puts her hand on my knee. "You're doing it, Jen. This will be tough, but you don't have to do it alone. You'll have nursing help. We'll get through it."

I believe her, because she's Grace and only because of that. She gives me what I need to face what's ahead and to give Rob, give us, what we wish — his death in our bed, in our home. Months of trust undergirding me in this moment allow me to believe her words.

Thanks, Grace, I think, but I can't speak. If I speak, the deluge will come. I walk her to the door. "Bye, Grace."

A mix of tears and shock is mingling in my eyes and heart. This is what we've known would come, but it feels almost unreal that it's here. Yet it's real enough. Rob's struggle up the stairs is real. Grace's quiet, serious energy watching him was real.

"Bye, Jen," she says, softly, tenderly.

She leaves. I close the door. The tears come, and I lean against the door, unable to halt the wailing pouring from my heart. The dam has burst, and we are here. He's dying.

How can we have come this far, through the delirium, the methadone switch, without having to admit Rob to hospital to now have to take him there, to a hospital bed? But can I do this? Can I really keep him home? How are we going to keep the downstairs quiet enough for him, with the kids and his family around? But I have to do it somehow.

I realize I have to check on Rob. I go upstairs, and he's sleeping quietly. Grace's book is still in my hand. Not something I could have faced reading until this very moment. I pick it up and start reading. It is all new information, and I read and read and read. Bed baths, mouth care, breathing changes, and again the steep learning curve sets in.

There may be some clues in here; we've done the impossible so many times. I have to find the possible way for Rob to die at home. This book is the right gift in the right moment, it has in it what I need. The steps. The tasks and the knowledge of what to look for. We will do it. Rob will make sure we do this at home.

Monday 13 September 2010
E-mail from Jen to Grace

> *Thanks for the visit and the chat today. I needed you today and as always you were right there.*
>
> *I've been leafing through the book you left me. I'm wondering about the bed, the stairs, etc. What do you see when people are in the community?*
>
> *Does everyone get a hospital bed? Clearly that would end our sleeping next to each other. I'm sure that's what every Occupational Therapist would recommend, but wondering what your experience is (and I'm sensing you will say "it's individual, a personal choice, and whatever becomes practical at the time"). I would like to know what actual real 'live dying patients' do when they still want to be in bed with their spouse?*
>
> *Also, wondering your thoughts about location. We have talked about converting the dining room to a bedroom when he can't do stairs anymore, but for Rob that's such a 'last step'. What do people do in the meantime? Does everyone 'move downstairs'? Do people ever 'rent' stair lifts? Just wondering what your experience is, and to be honest looking for your opinion on where you think we may need to go.*
>
> *He was still a bit mixed up when you left, is sleeping now, will see where the evening takes us.*
>
> *Jen*

CHAPTER 19

The Last Hurdle

∽

Tuesday 14 September 2010
E-mail from Jen to Grace

> *Hi Grace,*
>
> *So Rob woke up confused again today. Can't find his words, having trouble describing symptoms, but I gather he has no pain.*
>
> *Just wondering, reading this book you gave me, it looks as though he has many symptoms of 'superior vena cava syndrome' (I have no idea what that is but the list of symptoms matches very closely). Not sure if there's anything new to be done about that, but wondering.*
>
> *I'm sitting here with him in our room, he's snoozing. Let me know if there's anything else you think I should be doing.*
>
> *Thanks,*
>
> *Jen*

Tuesday 14 September 2010
E-mail from Jen to Helen

> *Hi Helen,*
>
> *So can you sense the tidal wave? Rob's had a hell of a couple days; he's been confused, more pain. This morning I was leafing*

through a book Grace left for me. The book is a how to guide for care-givers of end of life patients, so pretty clear message in that. Anyway, there was a section on "things to watch out for" which included spinal cord compression, etc. and there was something called "superior vena cava syndrome"(SVCO), of which Rob had all but one of the symptoms. This means there is a huge clot in a vein leading to his heart and it could mean a sudden death.

I just wrote Grace, giving her an update on today and asked if that could be something we should look at. Long story short; the palliative care doctor called an hour later. She and Grace had spoken, and she indicated she had suspected a possible SVCO a few days ago when she saw Rob based on some of his symptoms. She wants to book Rob for a C.T. scan to see if he has an SVCO, which apparently could be treated with radiation and if not could result in an abrupt cardiac event, and death. It also may explain Rob's symptoms of the last two days.

She has put in a referral to a radiation oncologist, and booked him for a C.T. scan at eight thirty Friday morning in Woodstock, and changed some meds to hopefully get him through the next few days until they sort out what's happening.

When Rob's delirium started to clear this evening he said he thought this morning may have been the end. I did as well, but a little extra pain medication, and he's rallied. And, as of this moment, would like to proceed with the C.T scan and radiation if possible. So be it. We'll see if he's still here Friday.

I found myself telling him this morning he could go if he needed to, that I would miss him terribly, and please make sure you find me when you're on the other side. I asked him in the midst of his confusion if he thought he was done. He looked so clear for a second, looked right into me "not yet".

Tonight he seems more stable and is eating and drinking, which he wasn't this morning. The roller coaster peaks and valleys are getting very close together.

Take care. I hope you can hold us in your thoughts tonight.

Jen

Tuesday 14 September 2010
E-mail from Helen to Jen

> *I will Jen, I'm really with you. You are a brave woman reading your words saying to Rob you will let him go if he needs to go. Huge gift of love that. One of the most pure, I think.*
> *Holding up your heart, Rob and your family.*
> *Helen*

Wednesday 15 September 2010
E-mail from Jen to Grace

> *Hi Grace,*
> *So, you'll be aware of all this, but e-mailing you seems to keep me grounded. Dr. Fryer is now going looking for an SVCO, she's trying to arrange a C.T. scan. She's put a referral to radiation oncology and it sounds like if it is an SVCO, that radiation could be an option to treat.*
> *We have a new lazy boy lift chair in the living room. My parents bought it used on Kijiji from a widower, only used for three weeks before his wife died, looks brand new. Rob loves it and so does my back.*
> *I hope we get more than three weeks out of it.*
> *Take care,*
> *Jen*

Thursday 16 September 2010
E-mail from Jen to Grace

> *Hi Grace,*
> *We spent the morning with the United Church minister, planning Rob's funeral. It was a tough morning, but that weight seems to be lifted.*
> *We're talking about raised toilet seats this morning, any sugges-*

tions at the best version? Do you know if I can get that through CCAC? Trying to think of what we can do to make life easier for him.
Talk soon,
Jen

Thursday 16 September 2010
Phone Call from Dr. Fryer

Jen

"HI, JEN, I'VE SPOKEN TO GRACE, and I've arranged for a CT scan at Woodstock Hospital tomorrow at eight in the morning," Dr. Fryer informs me.

"I'll talk to Rob about it. Thanks for arranging this. I have to go now." I hang up. I can't imagine getting Rob to a CT scan at eight in the morning tomorrow. He is so exhausted, and I know he's dying.

I walk into the living-room.

Rob is resting on the lift chair that we just obtained for him. He can no longer get off the couch on his own. He looks terribly sick.

"I've just talked to the doctor. They need a CT scan in order to confirm an SVCO. If it turns out that you do have one, they can treat it at the cancer clinic with radiation. It sounds like five to ten days of radiation, once a day, every day."

Rob makes a face. "I don't like the sounds of that," he says.

I kneel down beside his chair and hold his hand. "This is completely your choice, and only you know what to do here. The only reason we go for the CT scan is if you would then choose to carry on and have the radiation. You can also choose to not have the CT scan, stay home, and relax on your new lift chair. If it is an SVCO and it's not treated, you could die very quickly. But," I pause, deep breath, "I think that's maybe where we're going anyway. If the SVCO doesn't finish things, the cancer will."

Rob looks at me and says, with his irrepressible humour, "Well, I do really like this lift chair!" Then, more seriously and slowly, holding my gaze, "I love you, Jen. I love my house. I just want to stay here with my family. I don't want to be travelling."

He pauses, and I can see he's really wrestling with this decision. There are so many layers of meaning to it. He looks at me and says, decisively, "I'm not having radiation."

We both know what this means.

Rob is very clear. It's just too hard on him to move anywhere. He's done. He's where he wants to be.

"OK. I'll call Grace and the doctor. No CT scan Friday morning."

"I love you. Jen."

"I love you too."

I know in this moment that he is going to die in the next few days. I know we've made the right choice. I expect that, CT scan or no CT scan, his body has finished. I can tell by looking at him. And he's ready to go. He's done fighting. He just wants to let go.

I feel relief in a way. It's been so difficult to help him to the last few appointments, and I've found myself thinking, "This is pancreatic cancer, we're in the end of life, why are we dragging him around anywhere?"

He's obviously come to the same point. He looks comfortable in his chair, and I just don't want to be the one to inflict anything other than comfort on him. Even if the treatment would mean an extra week or two. This battle is over. It's time.

I call Grace and the doctor and leave messages. I say the same thing to both of them, "I've just had a conversation with Rob about the CT scan scheduled for Friday. He has decided he's not interested in pursuing the CT scan or any subsequent radiation to treat a potential SVCO. We've shifted gears, and we need to just make sure he's comfortable and ready to go."

We've made peace with all possible eventualities and ways to die. So be it. We're ready.

I hang up. I feel like it's all happened so fast. I don't exactly know what's ahead of us, but I know I'm going to lose him. My mind is reeling. I can't lose him. I realize I have to prepare everyone — the children, his parents, his brothers. I realize that Rob and I have just realized he will die very soon, but no one else knows. And Rob's not going to be able to tell anybody. I have to do it.

I kneel next to him. I've so little time remaining with him. The whole year of this illness has flown by. I can't believe I'm going to lose him.

We've gone from "You're in a lot of pain and, yes, dying" to "You're dying." I am bringing Grace and the doctor up to speed. They aren't aware of how quickly Rob's body is letting go. We're there. I'm not sure they are yet.

Thursday 16 September 2010

Grace

"Fuck."

I say that to myself.

I've just received a phone message from Jen telling me they've talked and Rob has decided that he is not having the CT scan and not going to London for radiation. I know if he has an SVCO we can treat that. I have been anticipating that we'll treat it. When I receive this message, I know clearly this means he's done.

I'm very sad. For the most part with this cancer, it's a done deal. But still, when everything stops because the end is near, it's tough. It's just tough.

There is a life in their relationship that is so unique, so touching. Not every case touches you like this in this job. Death is a part of living, and it makes us embrace life and living. That's my more common experience. You accept the deaths that happen. Then there are a few that touch you that are remarkable. Jen and Rob have been one of those cases.

I feel a sense of failure, even though I know full well that is not rational. I always keep hoping for survival, until there is no hope, even for a short time. But now, there is nothing more to do. All the tricks up my sleeve for dealing with symptoms, for managing the side-effects of both cancer and treatments, are no longer of any use.

Rob has defeated the odds, and, emotionally, I've invested myself in supporting them in their death-defeating and living-against-the-odds journey. When someone lives against the odds, I keep investing and investing because they keep defying the statistics. It's the yin and yang of intellectual knowing of outcomes and the emotional experience of hope.

And here, I confront now the inevitable. The end of his trajectory has come. I have to lay down my desire to 'do more.' It's the letting go as a health care provider that's the hardest part of all.

We need the professional mantle that we carry to do this work. I try to hide my disappointment that Rob is now saying "No" to possible treatment. I know this shows how deeply I care. I have to hide it and wear the mantle. I see Jen and Rob have reached the end point. *They* are telling *me,* "No," and usually it is the other way around. Usually, we are telling people that they're at the end of all possibility for effective treatment.

We're the ones counselling them in their emotional turn around to accept that and embrace the end-of-life process. Now, Rob is the one who has identified the reality that he is dying, and Jen is fully supporting him. They aren't asking for — and they don't need — any more tricks up my sleeve They're telling us that it's over. How the tables turn. Now we're in a different road.

Ten Days in September

∽

Thursday 16 September 2010
E-mail from Jen to Helen

> *It's been a hell of a day.*
> *We met with the minister and have laid all ground work for a memorial service for Rob.*
> *Rob has had such a lot of pain; everything seems to be changing so quickly. After a tough discussion, he has elected to cancel the CT scan for tomorrow morning, acknowledging realistically that even if it did show an SVC obstruction, he doesn't have the energy to get to London to treat it with radiation. I believe he has made the right decision.*
> *The rain seems appropriate today, very stormy here, and very, very tender.*
> *Talk soon.*
> *Jen*

Thursday 16 September 2010
E-mail from Helen to Jen

Thanks for the update Jen. I was up early, around five again, so breathing, sending my heart energy to you all. It's like I'm right there or you're right here.

Can you get any friends to make soups for you for the coming week, food that's easy to go down that can be popped in the freezer to keep? You likely won't feel like eating for a long time to come so best not rely on the body cues to tell you to eat.

And I was thinking about the children and their involvement in this time. I am assuming Jack and Haley are with their dad right now? Do you think they need a time of goodbye, perhaps draw pictures for him for his 'journey' ahead, or something they can do for him from 'their world'? Again, the closeness and being part of the circle is often helpful for them, albeit briefly, rather than being one step removed and then just hearing that he's gone. Doesn't have to be long and drawn out.

Far from morbid, it often brings a place for the grief to be shared, which the younger children need to see, be part of, have a chance to feel themselves in a safe circle of love around their sadness and often it feels comforting and 'completing.'

I asked the 'grandmother' tree, as my native friends call it, in our back yard which has watched several native ceremonies there in the last year with my elder friends, to watch over Rob. I do believe, as the native wisdom teaches, that the life support system of the earth is deeply interconnected with us.

I offered tobacco and called on the web to send the prayers to Rob. A goldfinch showed up under the cedars when I got to those trees with the tobacco as well and then flew off, almost as a messenger. So, he's not alone in his inner journey. A deep peace was present in that moment. He's got the guides, whoever they are with him now. I sense you're not alone.

Staying close.
Helen

Thursday 16 September 2010

Jen

ROB HAS BEEN IN BED since Thursday night, two days now. The last two days the house has been empty. Ben is seeing friends, Jessica's at university, and my parents have the kids. It's been really good to have just the two of us in the house. By now, I've taken over all personal care of Rob, and I'm so glad Grace gave me the book, which I've now read two or three times, cover to cover.

I've heard from Grace that she and Dr. Fryer are supposed to arrive at our house today. That's never happened before; we've never had both of them in the same day. And I realize I'm not waiting for any information or for them to tell us anything I don't know.

Rob is taking a small amount of food in bed on a tray. He is curious: "I wonder why both of them are coming. I feel very important! And on a weekend!"

I notice, with heartache, how weak he is, but how hard he's trying to still make light of what is happening, buffering the stark truth of it, for me. Then he adds, sincerely, thinking of others, as is his way, "I hope I'm not ruining their weekend plans."

Grace arrives. I bring her upstairs. I know that in three days Rob has declined significantly, and I watch her to see her reaction. She sits down in a chair in the corner. She has a very different way of being today. She's lost her saltiness, and tenderness comes over her as she says "Hi" to Rob.

He quietly acknowledges her hello.

"Dr. Fryer is held up in Toronto and can't make it here," she says.

Rob nods, understanding. He looks puffy, flushed, and sweaty, with no energy at all, but he's very calm. There's no sense of fear or pain. He looks very comfortable. He's engaging Grace with his quiet, steady way as she asks him about how he's doing and making some medication suggestions, cutting things out he doesn't need at this point.

I ask her, "We want to know how long you think he's got? Rob doesn't want a big bedside vigil that's going to go on for weeks."

Grace responds, slowly, "Well, as I sit here, I see a man who is still eating and taking drink. Rob, you're still very lucid, aware of your surroundings and interactive, so I certainly don't think we're down to the last few hours." She adds, "I also don't think you're going to see weeks, likely several days."

"We'll start to think about how we'll call people in then," I respond, my brain already working.

"We'll call the home visiting nurse, and she should start coming in at least once a day," Grace affirms. "You might want to introduce medications by subcutaneous injection rather than orally, and I think we just need more eyes on you now, Rob."

She is rallying the troops. We go over a few more details, and our visit ends.

"Goodbye, Rob," she says, gently.

"Bye," he responds, just as gently.

I walk her back downstairs. She says, "I think you should call Jessica home, and you probably should be telling her professors that she's going to be off for a bit." Grace, thinking of all the dimensions, as is her gift. "And," she adds, "I don't think you should be alone in the house in case he falls, you'd need someone to help you."

"OK. I'll make sure Ben starts staying home," I reply. I become aware of the logistics ahead for safety. I realize that when I tell Ben this, it is going to shift things radically. My time alone with Rob in the house is going to come to an end forever. I feel a wave of sadness flood through me. I know this is how it has to be. I have to let go of my imagining I'd be quietly alone with Rob as he slipped away by my side.

"Good plan, Jen. Get Jessica home and make sure Ben is home as well. Sounds good," Grace affirms. Then adds, putting her hand gently on my shoulder, "Hang in there. I'm only a phone call away."

She leaves, and I go back upstairs. I have to say goodbye to our cocoon of the last few days in the sanctuary of our bedroom, with Rob comfortable. All the care I've given him has developed an even greater tenderness between us. It's been sacred time. And now it will change.

Saturday 18 September 2010
E-mail from Jen to Grace

Hi Grace,

I'm sorry I couldn't talk to you longer today at the end of the visit. I do need some help planning out what other help I'll need. We have lots of offers; I just need to sort out what we'll need when. So far I've been fine on my own and have cherished the time together with Rob. But, I realize I will need more support at some point soon so I'll think on that. One day at a time.

Rob's had a good evening; sat and chatted with Ben and I about his grandma. I asked him who his angel would be to help him through and that sparked the conversation. Rob's pain has been manageable, not confused.

I did a bed bath, gave him a shave, changed the sheets; nurse Jen. He looks and smells much better. Has that distinctive cancer breath, you must know what I mean. I don't know what it is, liver I'm guessing, but I smell it all the time at the London Regional Cancer Program, very distinctive, not terrible just distinctive. It's new in the past week.

Talk soon. I'll give you an update after the nurse comes.

Thanks as always for today. I am sorry we had to eat into your weekend.

Jen

Saturday 18 September 2010
E-mail from Jen to Helen

Hi Helen,

I was up at five in the morning with Rob, but slept all night next to him before that. Well, I didn't sleep all that time, awake listening.

Rob spent time last night with Ben; saying he felt he's lived a good life, has no regrets, never had a bucket list, just wanted to spend time with all of us, which he has. It was hard for us all.

Jessica has been apprised of things more directly this morning and I said following the appointment today with the doctor and Grace I would call her with a plan, and bring her home to be with her dad. She sounded numb.

I was thinking the same of Jack and Haley this morning. I would like them to say goodbye. They are with Dave.

I feel calm here the past two days; it's been mostly Rob and I, just here in our room, lying next to him as he sleeps. I have almost finished reading "On Grief and Grieving" by Elisabeth Kubler-Ross. I needed to pick that up when I did. There is a section on angels, call them what you will, but I find myself asking Rob to see if he can find his angel and also know that one day he will be mine.

Take care. I will stay in close touch.

Jen

Sunday 19 September 2010
E-mail from Helen to Jen

Hi Jen,

It's a very sacred time. You are without doubt a soul guide with him for him as he has been for you. Your presence is a deeply significant part of this process in some way. The two of you have been forming a bond so deep, so real that I suspect it already transcends the time and space of this visible realm. Your 'co-mingling' of your love is strengthening something invisible and eternal between you.

I so feel you are not alone in that room and home of yours. I've asked my elder friends to say prayers for Rob and you as well and they are.

Blessings in this sacred, painful, heart wrenching, spirit-filled time.

Helen

Monday 20 September 2010
E-mail from Jen to Grace

Hi Grace,

I phoned England, the phone call to Rob's mum was hard. I gave
her an update last night, and another one today, all at Rob's instruc-
tion. Rob was able to speak to her for a minute, which was heartbreaking for her I'm sure. She says she will have a flight probably
Wednesday. I wonder if he might be gone by then. I didn't say that to
her, just said it was time for her to come.

Jen

Monday 20 September 2010
E-mail from Jen to Grace

Hi Grace,

How long could this go on for?

My kids came by with my mom after school to say goodbye. She
told them Rob might be dying tonight and they both wanted to see
him. He opened his eyes and hugged them and said he loved them.
I'm glad they saw him. We were all here in the room, everybody. It
was hardest for Rob I think, precious time in his life.

We are in the final hours now I think, I've told him to let go and
I think he's trying. Tough body though. Jack has refused to leave the
house with my mom, so both kids are downstairs with her, quiet. I
have asked her to please get them to her house, she's trying.

Into another long night.

Isn't today the last day of summer?

Jen

Monday 20 September 2010
E-mail from Grace to Jen

> *Dear Jen,*
> *You have prepared them well. Your mom will be able to support in being where it is best for them to be. You and Rob have done this for them. If they are there that is ok. The visiting nurse will help you with them. They might not want to be there when the funeral home comes but this seems to be proceeding very gently and perhaps they are meant to be there. Hang in there. Trust yourself. Trust the work you and Rob have gallantly laid before you.*
> *God Bless.*
> *Grace*

Monday 20 September 2010

Jen

I'VE BEEN LYING NEXT TO ROB for the past several hours in our bed. I've wondered what this will be like for the past year. In many ways, it's what I'd hoped for in so much as we're home. I have my hand on his chest, tracking his heartbeat.

"I'm right here with you," I whisper to Rob. "It's time for you to go. I know you'll find me on the other side. I know you'll always be with me. I love you. I know you love me, but now it's time for you to go."

I repeat it over and over, like a mantra, in his ear. I know he hears me. Sometimes, he says, "I love you." Sometimes, he says, "I want to go." Sometimes, he says, "I know."

He seems totally peaceful as I tell him to let go. This becomes my whispered message to him, over and over, this week of his dying.

Monday 20 September 2010
E-mail from Jen to Helen

> *I think we're in the final hours. Ben and Jessica are here. Family has been called, it is peaceful, and he is comfortable. I would like you to come if at all possible sometime afterwards before the funeral.*
> *Jen*

Monday 20 September 2010
E-mail from Helen to Jen

> *Hi Jen,*
> *Will be there in spirit through this and happy to come and visit you after. Absolutely. I'm glad it's peaceful. May you be surrounded by all the angels, all the guides and all the conscious beings and ancestors who are part of this journey with you.*
> *Holding you all very closely and tenderly.*
> *Helen*

Monday 20 September 2010
E-mail from Jen to Helen

> *Hi Helen,*
> *The parallels between birth and death are so apparent right now; the waiting, the anticipation, the prayer for safe delivery, the pain, the rhythm of breathing and contraction changing over time. The family waiting, the hushed voices, the nurses' tidy ways. You have talked about this, but I never understood. Even the wish of "please let this be over, it's time" that I remember feeling when I was in labour with Jack, and the demand of patience from nature's timetable.*
> *The children are staying here, downstairs with my mom. Your e-mail and one from Grace echoing the same has let me let it happen.*
> *Jen*

Monday 20 September 2010
E-mail from Helen to Jen

Hi Jen,
    There is a very 'altered state' feeling to this whole day. I really want you to know that I am deeply convinced that there is a whole weaving happening around this timing and the threads between the visible and invisible.
    My children know that we are praying for Rob tonight and they are holding Jack and Haley in their little hearts particularly. It's very touching. The circle is wide and close.
    If your children need to stay, let them. They may need to be close and they don't have to be right there in the room. 'Death' is only fearful if we as adults make it so. Trust their asking, trust their guidance. They will know where they need to be. Death is a community event, part of the circle. They may be helping him transition simply by being there downstairs, who knows.
    Blessings.
    Helen

Monday 20 September 2010
E-mail from Helen to Jen

Hi Jen,
    I gathered with my native friends tonight, around the fire for their special ceremony. I wanted to just share with you that an image of Rob, flashed into my mind's eye, he was huge! Sort of like an archangel huge. Again, almost like I was seeing his energy body and it was blue and purple-ish.
    It is what I imagine the 'rainbow body' that buddhists talk about, would look like. I wonder if sometimes the 'leaving the body' takes time and that it almost might be like a butterfly, stretching out of the cocoon, five times larger than its encasement and perhaps a time of 'strengthening' before leaving finally. It's not the first time I've felt

the leaving of the body may take more than just a moment but be a process.

I stood up and shared about you and Rob, briefly and that I was praying for you tonight. The fire flared and Dan, the elder, looked up and said, "He's here." I felt Rob so strongly that I talked 'to' him instead of praying 'for' him. It felt quite real.

Courageous woman that you are, Jen. Fearlessly walking this moment by moment. Staying present, as you have all along, and I mean really, really present. Your children are absorbing something very important and real through you in this. You are the one to be held after Rob's journey is over on this side of real. May whatever you need to keep you surrounded by a great circle of love keep finding you.

Another night, another darkness. May he find his way in the perfect moment.

Breathing with ...

Helen

Tuesday 21 September 2010
E-mail from Jen to Helen

Hi Helen,

We are still on this road. Rob is hanging on for something, I don't know, maybe it's his parents who arrive tonight. He is quite sedated today; they ordered something to relax him, he's been getting agitated.

Rob is peaceful. His body is dying and changing in appearance, but Rob is peaceful.

Thanks,

Jen

Tuesday 21 September 2010
E-mail from Helen to Jen

Hi Jen,
*   And one more thought... take as much time as you need with*
his 'body' when he does finally go. You don't need to rush him out
the door. The Irish tradition would 'wake' the person for at least a
day and night and traditionally it used to be a week in the house.
*   Trust your needs in this too and don't let other needs, rules, or*
perceived pressures steer you away from what you need. Trust your
gut, if he looks peaceful as to whether you want the children to see
his body too. It demystifies 'death' again for them if it feels right.
*   When he leaves the house though, that is something, perhaps,*
to not let them witness. Expect that to be a very difficult moment
for yourself and have support for that time, your mom perhaps.
*   Blessings to you all in whatever ways you need them now.*
*   Helen*

Wednesday 22 September 2010
E-mail from Jen to Grace

Hi Grace,
*   Another long night. Rob's parents arrived just before midnight;*
he was responsive but then became agitated after seeing them, had
rattly shallow breathing all night. I had everybody here in my room
until four in the morning. Not much sleep last night.
*   This morning breathing is not as rattly, not as shallow, and talking*
(little loopy) a bit to me, Jessica and Ben. Now he's asleep.
*   Dr. Fryer is coming to see him today.*
*   I told him to go, he says he wants to, he's trying. The visiting nurse*
is here now, she's baffled. No idea how long this may go on for. I wish
his body would stop.
*   That's today*
*   Jen*

Wednesday 22 September 2010
Home Visit from Dr. Fryer

Jen

IT'S MID-AFTERNOON, and there's a light knock on our bedroom door. My Mom is there and tells me that Dr. Fryer has arrived. The doctor comes in, carrying a plate with a bun on it, and says, "Your Mom has asked me to give this to you and make sure you eat it! She's worried about you. She says you haven't slept and you haven't eaten in days. I've told her that this is where you need to be. So she asked me to give you this bun."

"Well," I reply, "she's right. I haven't slept more than a few minutes on and off in the past seventy-two hours. But I'm OK. "

I realize as I tell her this that I am calculating how long it's actually been, and I can't believe I've been awake this long. I feel tiredness but not exhaustion, and I know that I absolutely will just keep going as long as I need to. I am receiving energy from somewhere for this journey with Rob into his death.

The last three or four days I have had a very unusual experience. It is almost like an altered state. I've felt completely at one with Rob in every possible way, as if we're sharing one body, one mind, one heartbeat. I have been able to feel what he's feeling.

I feel when he needs meds and exactly which one he needs. It's always right at the time when he needs the dose, which my look at a clock or chart confirms. And I also know intuitively when he needs extra meds between scheduled doses. As I lie next to him, I will have a sensation that he is beginning to experience pain or nausea, and even before he begins to stir I'm reaching for the medicine.

I can't understand how this is happening, but it is. I think back and realize that when he was in the opioid-induced delirium, last month, I had been preparing for this moment. It taught me to rely purely on my intuition, because his verbal feedback was totally unreliable. Through that time, we strengthened a flow of silent communication back and forth, beyond words, and I have now completely tuned into it.

At this point, Rob appears to be asleep. Jessica and Ben leave the room, so it's just Dr. Fryer, Rob, and I. I go up to Rob and sit on the bed next to him, touching his face very slightly, "Hi, sweetheart. Dr. Fryer's here to see you."

His eyes flicker open, and the doctor moves over to him and lightly puts her hand on his shoulder: "Hi, Rob. How are you doing?"

"OK," he replies.

"Are you having any pain?"

"No pain," he says, almost inaudibly.

"Are you comfortable?"

"Yes," he whispers.

She looks at him, I notice, with great tenderness. "Is there anything more you need to do, Rob?"

I wonder what she's asking. It's a strange question.

Rob becomes a little more alert and responds, "No. I'm all done." Then he continues, "I'm ready to go home. It's time for me to go."

"You can go, Rob, anytime you want," she quietly affirms. "Your family is here. They've all said goodbye, and there's nothing more you have to wait for. You can go whenever you want."

He replies, "That's good. That's good." He starts to drift off. Dr. Fryer moves away from the bed and turns to start talking to me. Just then Rob interjects in a stronger voice, "How do you think I'm doing?"

I wonder how much of this he is actually following. He seems a bit confused. What is the physician supposed to say to this question? He's dying ...

She walks back over to the bed, "Well, it seems like you're comfortable. You've said your goodbyes; you're here in your home, just as you wanted. I think you're doing just great. Is there anything you need?"

She is so good with us in this. Everything she's saying is so fitting. I can tell she's seen many people die before.

Rob replies, "I'd really like some Kendal Mint Cake."

I have no idea what Rob is talking about! I assume it's one of his childhood English treats. I'll have to ask his family. I lean into him and say, "Sweetheart, I don't think you can even swallow cake right now." I feel so bad that I can't fulfil his wish, but he just can't take solids at all.

The doctor leans over him and says, "Well, Rob, maybe we could get you a little bit of mint ice-cream. Would that be OK?"

I feel rescue and great relief.

Rob nods slightly, "Yes ... that would be good ... ice-cream ..." he says, smiling and smacking his lips lightly. Clearly, this is a very good idea!

I lean out of the bedroom door and ask Jessica if she can find a spoonful of ice-cream and a Q-tip to feed her father with. I go back into the bedroom. Rob has drifted back into sleep again.

Dr. Fryer and I stand at the door a few feet away from Rob, and she turns and looks right at me, saying, "You've done a wonderful job, Jen. He's comfortable, he's in no pain, and he seems very content. This is exactly where he wanted to be. In his home, in his own bed, with you looking after him. I can't imagine a greater gift."

I share with her my last, lurking concern, "Is there anything that could happen now that would change his being able to stay here? Is there any reason that we'd have to move him out of the house?"

She pauses and takes a big breath and smiles, "No. He will stay in the house. We are prepared for every eventuality, I can't think of any possible reason why he would have to leave. You've done it, Jen."

I feel a huge flood of relief. My biggest fear is that Rob will die in a hospital bed somewhere other than here. She's alleviated even my lesser fear of having him downstairs in the middle of our living-room, in a hospital bed. I breathe out slowly. I'm so grateful that he's dying at home, dying in his own bed, and dying with me beside him. It's all happened as we'd hoped.

I tell the physician about Jack and Haley's coming in two days ago to say goodbye to him. As I'm telling her about Rob's hugging them and saying goodbye, I notice her eyes are welling up with tears.

"Both of you have done a wonderful job preparing your children," she affirms. "You have prepared well for all of this."

"Do you have any sense of how much longer this will go on for?" I figure she, of anyone, having seen him now, with her expertise, will have the best guess.

"At this point, the timing will be completely up to Rob. He's in charge."

Again, I don't receive an answer. This is nature's timetable. The mystery of death.

"OK," I say.

Dr. Fryer hugs me, which she has never done before. "Take care of yourself. This will be over soon." And then she leaves.

Wednesday 22 September 2010
E-mail from Jen to Helen

Hi Helen,
Rob's body is still here, he wants to go, and Dr. Fryer, who came today said it could be anytime, or it could go for many days.
His parents arrived last night. His breathing was rattly last night. We all thought that was it, but into the morning we came, and his breathing stopped rattling.
Today he's been hallucinating a little, first about a bear in the back garden. There is meaning about bears, about transitions I believe. He also was talking about chocolate, and ice cream, and cars, and Liverpool. This morning when it was just us at about six in the morning he said: "On this my last day it's just me."
"I'm here with you, sweetheart," I said.
"I know you are. And I'm with you. I'll always be with you."
I am upstairs in our sanctuary bedroom with Rob.
Into another long night we go.
Jen

Wednesday 22 September 2010
E-mail from Helen to Jen

Hi Jen,
Going into the night with you, still holding you all very closely.
Now ice cream and Liverpool, no idea what the deep meanings of those are! But I'm sure glad he got to taste some!
Today the image in my mind's eye of Rob changed. He took on more colours in his huge warrior like energy body. As if it's getting stronger. Weird. I'm not prone to visions but I believe somehow Rob's energy body is strengthening through this 'in between' process.
Holding you energetically and the children, and Rob, as you hold him and all that's going on there.
Helen

Wednesday 22 September 2010
E-mail from Jen to Helen

Hi Helen,

I feel like he is in between. I know the sadness and sorrow and ache will come, but right now I feel like I want him to go because I know he's not all here anymore. And his poor, poor body, it is hard to see a physical body break when it was so active and alive and held me close so often. His edema is dissipating as this decline happens and left behind are wasted muscles of once strong arms, legs, and hands that healed so many other broken bodies. They look so bony. It's time for him to go.

I so hope and beg and pray that I will be able to sense Rob somehow later on. I will miss him so, I do already.

My children are incredible, they have been here this whole time and are there waiting to hug me when I steal a five minute break downstairs.

You have said all along that we were teaching them so much through this, but I wasn't sure I bought it. But I see how kids are so real and honest and resilient. They have seemed to just resent the fact that I need to spend less time with them, until this week. They are amazing. And yes, learning so much.

Haley spent this evening telling me all about butterflies, which she is learning about at school, "did you know mummy, it's a chrysalis, not a cocoon, only moths have cocoons, and it takes ten days for the butterfly to come out, and then its wings dry off, and then it eats the chrysalis to give it strength to fly.

I told her your 'story' about butterflies and how it can be compared to how a body dies and becomes an angel (Haley's words). She liked it.

Into the night we go.

Jen

Wednesday 22 September 2010
E-mail from Jen to Grace

Hi Grace,
A long day. My mom has dealt with all things downstairs.
Rob's had much more agitated spells today and has spoken a lot on and off, but much of it hallucinations about cars, chocolate, boxing, nice things.
Rob's mum let him know today that his twin brother Malcolm is flying in tomorrow evening. One more thing that I imagine he will wait for.
Grace I know you're going out of town, and I'm sure that after this is done, I will be in the midst of funerals etc and I will forget in all the commotion, but I wanted to thank you so much for all you have done. We are but one client on a busy caseload, but for us, your constant presence and availability, your tremendous clinical skill and unwavering commitment to Rob has kept me level and steady through a very long journey.
You have problem solved so much for us, you never once said "well guys that's tough, part of cancer, no solution". I always felt that you could magic up a solution to just about everything you did. Your openness to e-mails about all sorts has been invaluable to me and has often been the thread of sanity and hope that has delivered me through so many difficult days.
My mourning for the loss of my soul mate and partner started the day he was diagnosed, but you have so skillfully kept me focused on today, and we had so many wonderful todays this last year.
I know after Rob is gone I will also lose my connection to you, at least in this capacity, and I will mourn that as well. You have no idea how much you have meant to me this past thirteen months, thank you.
Into another night we go.
Take care,
Jen

Thursday 23 September 2010
E-mail from Grace to Jen

> **Hi Jen,**
> I hope u found Dr. Fryer's visit reassuring. Just want you to know, although I am 'away' tomorrow and Friday, I will still be connected. Take good care, you remain in my thoughts. One day at a time.
> Grace

Thursday 23 September 2010
E-mail from Jen to Grace

> Hi Grace,
> Thanks for the e-mails. I needed that one this morning early.
> Dr. Fryer's visit was reassuring, she said she thought his symptoms were exceptionally well controlled, that he looked comfortable, and that there would be no reason she could foresee that he would need to be moved or die anywhere other than here.
> I feel very proud I've been able to do this for him, it's what he wanted. He does look comfortable. He's been smiling in his sleep all morning.
> I slept from eleven to four, and then from four-thirty to six, which is more than I have since last Thursday. So I feel better. He seems much less rousable today, though still responds if I whisper right in his ear that I love him. He says "I love you" or "perfect" or "I know". He's sleep talking a bit too, mumbling bits of conversations, it's been entertaining.
> I hope you enjoy your time away.
> Thanks for everything grace. I'll keep in touch.
> Jen

Friday 24 September 2010
E-mail from Grace to Jen

Hi Jen,
 Hope you're hanging in. Malcolm's arrival certainly adds a new dimension.
 How are your little ones doing? Such a terribly long week for every one of you.
 Thinkin' 'bout ya'.
 Grace

Friday 24 September 2010
E-mail from Jen to Grace

Hi Grace,
 We had a night of extremely loud, gurgly, rattly breathing following Malcolm's arrival. Malcolm's a day behind on the "say goodbye" message. I'll need to talk to Malcolm sometime today about telling Rob from himself that it's ok for Rob to go. They're identical twins so on some level, I think Malcolm has to tell Rob that too.
 I think he's still here for Malcolm's sake, to let Malcolm come to terms. That sounds crazy I'm sure, but it is such a typical Rob thing to do, and unresponsive or not, I think that's his plan.
 He really needs to go. I was up until five in the morning listening to the loud breathing waiting for him to go, but he didn't. This is really tough.
 Thanks for checking in.
 Jen

Saturday 25 September 2010, 3:26 a.m.
E-mail from Jen to Grace and Helen

> *He's gone.*
> *We had his parents, his twin brother Malcolm, and Ben and Jessica all in the room for eleven hours of cheyne-stoking. At one thirty a.m. they all left and Ben stayed in the room so that Ben and I could reposition him and do mouth drops.*
> *Then Ben left for a moment and I sat on the bed next to him. I took Rob's hand and I said, "It's just me and thee, sweety."*
> *In that minute that it was just us, he died.*
> *Now the hard part starts.*

Saturday 25 September 2010
Final Rob Update

I'm writing to let everyone know that Rob passed away last night in the wee hours of morning today, Saturday. He died peacefully, with his mum and dad, his children Ben and Jessica, his twin brother Malcolm, and me all at his side. He died exactly how he wanted, at home, in his own bed, surrounded by his loved ones. He had no pain, and was completely comfortable in his last days, reminiscing about good times in his life; physio, sports, ice cream and chocolate.

Rob's battle was such a courageous one that has brought together so many people. Throughout the almost fourteen months of his illness he lived life to the fullest, day by day, enjoying every minute he had, never ever complaining, always finding the positive. Just the way he lived his life. The hole he has left in our hearts will never ever be filled. If I know Rob he will find a way to continue to be with us. Funeral details will follow.

Jen

_____

Epilogue:

How Do I Do This Alone?

Saturday 25 September 2010

Helen

I AM SITTING at my computer, tears spilling in surprising sobs, at Jen's e-mail. It has caught me off guard — the sense of loss I'm feeling. It's not as if I wasn't anticipating this moment. In fact, I have been, from the moment I met them. But now, after the year-long 'death walk' we've shared, which turned into one of the most incredible and life-affirming experiences I've witnessed and been part of, now I find the loss of this man very grieving.

He has changed my perspective on what is possible about living and, particularly, living with cancer. He has shown me, unequivocally, that it can in fact totally transform one's relationship with life and death, and he became a living testament that it can. He embodied something very powerful about hope and love. It's been a journey that has changed many, many people, and my tears show the truth of how much Rob has changed me, too. I realize his quiet and fearless presence has been a potent medicine for me. I realize, with these unbidden tears, that I will miss him.

And how will Jen walk the road ahead? How does a woman who has lost her great beloved after six glorious years of expanding love live alone, without him beside her? How will she navigate the gaping hole, parenting her children and his, without him? Many people have had to walk this road, yet there is no formula. Not only does she have to face the anguish of her grief, but she also has to become a single working parent, a single householder of a home into which they had poured tremendous love — all in one fell swoop.

'Treacherous' is a word that comes to mind for this kind of grief journey. Treacherous, and with no guarantees that a person can make it through to any place beyond the heartache. Possible, but no guarantees.

How will Jen do this?

I truly have no idea.

Saturday 25 September 2010

Grace

JEN'S NEWS OF ROB'S DEATH comes to me in a hotel room in Windsor, Ontario, where I have travelled to attend the wedding of the daughter of a dear friend (Betti). I open the e-mail first thing on waking and feel surprise at how much the finality of Rob's death surprises me. In unfamiliar surroundings, I find it strangely surreal. I warn families all the time of the 'shock' that the finality of death brings ... regardless of preparation, regardless of anticipatory grieving.

This juxtaposition of sadness with the joy of a wedding is not unfamiliar. Death all too often interrupts life's pleasures. I have come to appreciate this all too well in my new work as a nurse practitioner in palliative care in community.

My day is just beginning. Jen's message does not spoil it — rather it has given me an all-the-sweeter appreciation for the love Angie and Steve are about to celebrate, with everyone who loves them as witnesses. Angie's Dad, Matt, will not be there physically, but his presence will be a heartfelt experience for everyone he knew. I feel an incredible sense of thankfulness for the ability to share and witness that ultimate gift: Love.

Saturday 25 September 2010
E-mail from Jen to Grace and Helen

> *Hi there*
> *You've been to a lovely wedding today, Grace, so only read this when it won't spoil your day. No rush, just wanted to connect.*
> *I'm going to bed now, have had a bath and a sleeping pill and hoping it works. I've been put on antibiotics by Dr. Fryer for a raging throat infection that's likely been there a week and has engulfed my right tonsil, thank God for her.*
> *Today Rob's twin brother Malcolm has helped me with all the funeral arrangements, obituary writing and has done the entire phone calling. The funeral planning was not as bad as I thought. The guy was nice, he said he used to watch Rob and I walk to the post office every day, which is across from the funeral home.*
> *I've done very little. I keep feeling like I've forgotten to give Rob a medication, like I'm forgetting something vitally important. It's a horrible aching feeling. I've found myself trying to find quiet places in the house to cry, but people keep sneaking up on me and hugging me, or handing me hankies. My parents, Rob's parents, and Malcolm....they are not the people I want to be hugged by. I just want Rob.*
> *The bed is so big without him, his bedside table so empty of pill bottles. None of the furniture of the house is arranged how I want it, we rearranged it two weeks ago to accommodate a lift chair/easy boy that he only used for three days. Now it all looks unfamiliar, food tastes horrible, my back and neck ache from the past five days of lifting and turning Rob, and not sleeping.*
> *I'm just re-reading what I've just written and trying to sort out what I'm trying to say to you, I guess just that this feels so, so terrible, in every possible way. I feel so alone and I just wanted to connect with someone who knows me. I know there is no solution to this; I have to do this, this grief thing. But I feel too broken to do anything, let alone go through an emotional process that is supposedly eventually going to heal. Because right now I'm in too many pieces to*

*possibly ever heal from this. It's like breaking a jar full of sand; you
never get all the sand back, some of it slips through the cracks in the
floor or under the fridge and then it's gone.*

I can't believe how painful this is.

*I know other people grieve and have grieved, but what I had with
Rob was so unique, you know that, and maybe you will also know
how I can possibly do this, because I don't.*

Thanks for being on the receiving end of this.

Talk soon,

Jen

Tuesday 28 September 2010

Home Visit from Helen

Helen

I AM DRIVING ON MY WAY to see Jen. I really wonder how she's going to do
this journey without him. She's lost her love. She's lost her role of caring
for him, expressing her love in a thousand practical ways a day that caring
for someone with cancer provides. She's lost her good-humoured, quietly
present rock of support.

It has become very clear to me, reaching this moment in this year with
them, that I have always had a sense of what was ahead and where they
were heading. I too, it dawns on me, have relied, without even realizing
it, on Rob's steady and fearless living. Now, death has come. Now, Jen is
alone. Will life keep showing up for her? Every fibre in my bones believes
it *can*, but will she experience this? No guarantees. There are just never
any guarantees.

Bereavement can be a very rocky path, from which some people never
truly heal and reconnect with the land of the living. I've met some who
are as much in the grave as their loved ones, their lives now a hollow
shell. I notice I have some genuine concern for Jen. Is she going to make
it through this shattering? I also know that if she can't 'feel' Rob, now he's
died, that could be a worse shattering than the cancer diagnosis. And I

would be, in part, culpable for fostering that hope. Life after death. Who ever really knows? We just have our intuitions, the experiences of others sharing their experiences of seeing, hearing, feeling loved ones, teachings of various religious or indigenous traditions. It's still always a vast un-known.

I exit the highway with all these thoughts and more rattling in my heart and mind. I notice, for the first time in this whole year, I worry for Jen, really worry. I also know that for me to pull out of accompanying her in this process now would be another major loss for her.

Right now, the e-mails are still a lifeline, and I sense this must remain so for her, and that's an easy thing for me to give. They allow her to talk about how awful it is, a hundred times a day, if necessary. I know from personal experience how valuable another person, quietly witnessing our pain, staying present, is. In fact, it often makes the difference between healing through the crucible of suffering and experiencing total annihi-lation from the agony. My gut is saying it's not time for me to leave this journey yet.

I notice again the fields around me and feel the lifting of spirits that comes every time I leave the city as I turn onto the road leading to their village. I feel something. As I drive on, the feeling becomes more and more present. By the time I am less than one kilometre from their place, I can name what it is. It's Rob. Rob as I knew him in person. The essence of Rob. His presence. I can actually *feel* him.

My brain kicks into what my body is signalling and starts to think about whether people who have died 'stay local.' Is Rob staying near Jen? How come I couldn't feel him on the highway? I quiet my brain and just take in this strange experience. Occasionally, in sessions with people, I'll feel a presence of someone I worked closely with in sessions before they died. I have the sense they show up to help me sometimes. I've had such 'thoughts' but rarely speak them out loud.

Now, I'm unequivocally feeling the way Rob's presence would feel in my room. It's amazingly comforting. I know in that moment that Jen's going to be OK. Rob has not gone away. He'll see her through. Tears are running down my face. Relief and something else. Hope. It's real what I've said, hoped, and believed. Essence lives on. Ancestors through the veil are real. Something that has felt only tentative no longer does. Rob's done it. Rob's made it through and remains near his love. But I still wonder if this is real for Jen. In the end, that's the only thing that really matters.

I pull up to the house wiping my tears. Time to focus on Jen. A black cat leaps out of the side door, and immediately I feel again Rob's remarkable presence, but also his voice, a trace of his voice, in my head says, *Watch the cat.* I remember how many cultures think cats are able to see into the realms beyond death and mediate spirits from there to the living. Jen appears right next to the cat.

"Hi, Helen." Jen looks exhausted. Completely wrung out. I give her a big hug. We head into the couch where Rob used to sit. I sit where I sat the first time with the whole family, where his feet would have been. The black cat sits near us on the window sill. Watching. Jack and Haley are here, and this is the first time I'm meeting them. I give them the books I've brought, wonderful books for children, and one that works well for adults too, *Tear Soup.* Jack reads them as we start to talk, and Haley goes to Jen's Mom in the kitchen.

Jen describes how she's doing. Shares with me an intricate weaving of beauty and grief in the story of Rob's death and how deep their connection became that week of his dying. I firmly believe in the power of telling a story to foster healing. How many places welcome the story of a loved one's death? His death was peaceful, it happened to the best of Jen's ability to give him what he wanted and what they needed. And she was there for his last moment. Right with him.

"It's strange to use a word like 'beautiful' about death," she says. "But, in a way, there was something almost beautiful about how he died. He was so peaceful." Her tears are streaming as she tells me this. A 'beautiful death' doesn't take away the heartbreak, ever. It just means that regrets do not riddle the grieving.

She describes the grief. "It's just terrible, Helen. I can't eat, can't put anything in my mouth. I miss him so much." She looks like a rag doll, all her life energy drained. She stares at the floor, quietly asking, "How am I going to do this?"

How indeed? Same question they asked when they first met me. "How do we do this?" Except now she has a year of 'doing it.' And what a remarkable year. I have utterly no idea how she's going to navigate this part of the process. I see in my mind's eye a canyon with a very rickety bridge across it. The last year, with so many unexpected, life-affirming moments, suggests that she can. But grief can be a dangerous crossing.

"I don't know, Jen," I reply. "That was your question to me a year ago. You had no idea how you were going to live with death on your shoulder and believed it would just be bleak and terrible. But it wasn't only terrible. Life found you in so many ways. Life hasn't stopped with Rob dying. It will keep finding you." How, though, is the unknown, and there's nothing anyone can do to fill in that blank.

"I feel him, Helen." Jen says, looking at me.

"What do you notice?" I ask, with a sense of great relief and affirmation of my own inner sense of him around.

"He's all around me. I just feel him all round me. He's not gone. I feel his love like I always did when he was here."

Again, that sadness courses through her face, but within it a trace of steadiness. It is not the devastation of an annihilated hope. I sense the peaceful presence around her. Sad, yes, hollowed out, yes, raw, yes, but not annihilated.

"Well, I noticed driving here, about a kilometre from town, it was as if he was so present."

Jen looks at me with her tired, sad eyes. "Really?"

"Yes, very present."

The black cat moves from her spot. I watch her.

"You know, Shadow, the cat, has slept on Rob's side of the bed every night since he died," Jen comments. "Normally, she never hung out very much around us, but the week he was dying she sat on the window the whole time. Since he died, she sleeps next to me and purrs. When I'm crying, she puts a paw on me as if she's comforting me. Sometimes, I wonder if it's Rob."

This startles me. I was very willing to dismiss as pure fancy my fleeting thought of the cat as Rob's 'familiar' appearing at the door to greet me. There are limits to even my willingness to believe strange things. But sleeping in his spot now? Touching her when she's crying, when she's never hung out with Jen before? I feel goose bumps and a chill down my spine.

"I've brought some tobacco, Jen. It's a native tradition to offer tobacco as a prayer, and I brought some for the children as well. If they ever feel like they want to have a conversation with Rob, they can take the tobacco out to the garden and offer it and talk to him. It gives them something concrete to do, a tangible, simple ritual. That can help sometimes."

"Let's go for a walk round to the garden," Jen suggests. We head outside, Jack and Haley following us at a distance.

We stand under a big, old maple tree. "We're going to offer tobacco and say a prayer, which is a native tradition," I call to the children. "You're welcome to join us if you like, or not. Do whatever feels right for you." Jack stays nearby, but not too close. Haley stands next to Jen.

I offer the tobacco, giving thanks for the peaceful dying Rob had, and talk to him, "Well, Rob, I'm going to miss you a great deal. You've become a gift in my life just because of who you were when you were with us. Thanks for everything. I'm glad you're finding ways to stay connected."

I'm modelling something completely foreign to Jen and her children, but something that may help them to normalize talking to a person they love — something that many grieving people do for the rest of their lives, quietly. I'm encouraging her that it's not crazy. And the offering of tobacco is a simple act, embodying a connection with something beyond ourselves, be it earth, spirit, wind, ancestors, or whatever helps us to feel connection, not isolation.

Jen quietly puts her tobacco next to the tree, almost inaudibly whispering, "I miss you."

Shadow, the black cat, has joined us outside and is weaving her way towards us, right in this moment, to come and stand next to the tree.

"I feel him all around us," I quietly tell Jen. I feel something like a blanket of peaceful richness, with the ache of Jen's grief in the centre.

Jen nods in agreement. "Rob loved this tree. It was his favourite."

"It's a beautiful tree." I notice its wizened bark and knots. "You think about all this tree has weathered, Jen, all the storms it's lived through. You and Rob have been through an intense storm and weathered it. You metabolized cancer into love. This is what has come through as I've prepared the reflection for the funeral. Your love kept working with that cancer to keep creating love and life over and over, and you did it. Your relationship has alchemized the cancer into an incredible story of love. And love is life. Life will support you through this, just as it has through the last year, and just as it has supported the tree through all its storms."

We turn and head back into the house. Back into funeral planning and the intensely busy few days after someone has just died.

Friday 8 October 2010
Another Home Visit from Helen

Helen

I AM DRIVING to Jen's home for a second visit. The funeral was lovely, and many people came, even though it was a good distance from the city. There was beautiful sharing by Rob's twin brother about his younger years in England. Some funny stories, and more of Rob's quiet and powerful kindness. Stories of him at Parkwood Hospital by a close colleague, with the same thread running through them.

By the time I stood up, my thoughts had distilled into a simple essence: love — Jen and Rob's story is a love story. Love seeped into every moment of the fourteen months he lived with cancer. "They metabolized cancer into love."

Today, I am bringing chicken soup, hoping she will be able to eat something I made with care. I trust the body's wisdom to know how to heal, if it doesn't take on heavy demands to keep going and have a stiff upper lip. I don't worry about Jen's not eating. Still, I hope some chicken soup will help keep her strength and immunity up a little.

I've been watching her the last two weeks through her e-mails; again, she is just following her instincts, as we've often discussed. Cleaning, sleeping, staying in her pajamas, eating white bread, cleaning some more, getting her kids to school. Her e-mails have been an incredible description of the 'rawness' of her grief without self-pity or grasping her suffering around her like a blanket. Just her usual honesty and heartbreaking descriptions of her 'what is,' lacing it with humour on occasion, even now. And her incredible instincts. Along with cleaning, she's been knitting. Creating pattern and form instinctively in the midst of shattering chaos. It's truly amazing to me.

We're now at Thanksgiving. This is a tough weekend for anyone grieving any loss of a loved one. To add to the grief, today is also Jen's birthday. I'd asked her if she'd like a visit, knowing how difficult this holiday weekend might be, without Rob and with her children away at their father's and Jessica home for the weekend, also grieving. Jen had readily accepted the offer of soup and support.

As I round onto the road leading into the village at the exact same spot as the first time after Rob died, I have the same feeling — a peaceful sense of presence. It's the only way I can describe it. It fills with the 'sense of Rob' — it's not just any presence, as I feel in nature, it's Rob's particularity of presence. It strengthens, as it did before, as I head into the village and arrive at their home.

Jen greets me warmly at the door. She's still pale and tired, but I notice a settledness in her that wasn't there just before the funeral. It's been two weeks since Rob's death. The raw is now more cocooned in something else. As I go into the house, I notice how still it feels. It's as if the whole house is exhaling into a deep, deep stillness. It is not empty, however. I feel no emptiness at all. In fact, it feels full, life is still here.

Jen welcomes the chicken soup and a piece of felting art I'd created as Rob was dying. A collage of wool in autumn colours that seemed to weave my sense of his essence together as I'd experienced him. Last minute, as I was leaving my house, it seemed to need to come and be a gift to Jen today. I quickly wrapped it, and it came with me to her.

"I made this when Rob was dying. It's an image of his essence, I think. It's a circular mandala, the 'wholeness' at the heart of life. May it be heart-medicine somehow for you and your home."

Jen opens the hastily wrapped package, which delights her. "I know exactly where I'm going to put it — in our bedroom there's a spot on the wall above our bed. Thank you."

"Your house feels so peaceful, Jen," I comment. The stillness has crept into my awareness. I notice the polished floors and counters, fruits of her instinctive cleaning all the sickness out of the house.

"Yes, I imagine it's a lot different than the last time you came," she agrees. "It's my birthday today." Her tears well up. "It was six years ago that

Rob gave me this necklace." She touches the necklace around her neck, which, I notice, now has Rob's wedding ring on it as well. "It was the first gift he ever gave me."

She pauses and then adds, remembering with a sad smile, "You know, he mentioned my birthday the week he was dying. He said, 'I haven't bought you a birthday present yet.' I said, 'It's all right, sweetheart, you don't need to buy me anything.' Of course, he was bedridden by then. He said, 'I'll be with you on your birthday.' And I said, "Oh, Rob, you won't. That's three weeks away." He looked right at me and said, again, "Jen, I'll be with you on your birthday.' And I think he is, Helen. I really feel he is."

"What do you feel?" I ask, curious what it is she's sensing.

"He's all around. He's in the house. It's not a bad feeling. It's a wonderful feeling of him being all around me in the house. I hear echoes of his voice saying, 'I'm right here, I never left. I'm right here with you.' I think of all the times I just asked him to just stay, and he has. I really think he has. I feel him everywhere. I must sound crazy!"

I can feel the tears pricking my own eyes. It's such a bittersweet experience. He has gone. But something remains. And that something is holding Jen in a way that is preventing her from completely collapsing. It's enough, just enough. Rob's doing it. He's holding her.

"You're not crazy, Jen," I reassure her. "I feel him too, very much. I was wondering if the house would feel empty and his absence like a hole. I don't feel that. It feels full, so full of ... hard to name it, presence. Peacefulness ... love?"

"It doesn't make it any easier," Jen adds. "This is so, so hard."

"That's the bittersweet of it, so true. Nothing makes it easy," I agree. "Grief is so treacherous, Jen. Grief is very, very private, profoundly lonely. It's a wilderness of birth up in a cold cave on a mountain with rare help or contact with the outside world. It's really, really tricky to navigate, and no one can do it alone. You need lifelines of relationships that can just hold you in it, be present to the rawness, to the tears, to the grey. All of it.

"I'm staying in this with you, Jen. It's why Grace is still there for you and your family, your children. You just live it as you've lived this whole year, crying when you cry, comforting each other, getting on with the day, collapsing, again and again.

"Over time you learn how to navigate the loneliness, but the trick is to see it as you saw death, as the unwelcome guest who is now in permanent residence in your life that you have to work with somehow. In all of that, something healing is happening. It's invisible at first, but over time it will find its way through, and you'll realize the green shoots are pushing through the soil of the pain."

"The kids are struggling," Jen continues. A new, fresh sadness washes through her, visibly. "Jack is trying too hard to be a comfort for me. I feel terrible that he feels he has to take on this role of 'man of the house' and being there for me. He's only nine. Haley gets so upset every time she sees me cry, which is all the time. She says she feels so sad that I have to sleep in the bed by myself. Ben is just struggling with all of it. I don't have enough in me to provide the support that I'm sure he needs. Jessica is just drowning in university because, of course, university doesn't stop when your Dad dies. The little ones, though, I hate to say this out loud, but they're not doing as badly as I thought they might."

"You're all in this together, Jen. That's the important lifeline for the kids," I respond. And I believe it with every bone. Grief is not harmful. Avoidance of the truth and feelings is. Jen has never veered away from either.

I continue, "Everyone will have their own way through, no two of your journeys will look the same. One important thing you have to remember about the little ones is that they haven't lost the centre of their universe, they still have you.

"And grief can move through children in faster waves. We often assume grief will look the same in children as it does for us. When they cry, we think they're carrying it as we do, for as long as we do. But emotions move through children in waves that can pass, and they can be off playing happily after a moment of tears, and we're still carrying the grief of that moment for them, when they're long past it.

"You're teaching them how to live grief, Jen, as you have for a whole year. You let the waves move through and let them carry you out the other side, getting up, getting them to school, cleaning, knitting. Your instincts are guiding you because you're letting them, and so you're showing them how to live through grief by trusting those gut instincts that move you from one moment to the next. It's a powerful teaching you're giving them in how you're living this. And they're doing the same thing, because it's what you've taught them."

Jen nods. She can hear this because she's already lived this for many months. Now it's not a hypothetical possibility. Now it's living experience that I can just keep reflecting back to her. She's already done this. She's seen it bring life out of pain. Now she's applying trust from her own experience to the most difficult and anguishing part of all. Being alone without Rob.

"And the older ones will find their way in their own way. You can't do the grieving for everyone. They have to find how they heal through their own process. Let go of what's not yours to carry, or else it will bury you. Trust life will find them as it has you. Death will be everywhere for a long time, everywhere you look you'll see mirrors of the death your soul is feeling right now. Just remember to look up in those moments and see the birds, even if you can't feel life in the seeing, just see, just notice what is around you, and one day that bird will stir something in your heart, long buried, a feeling of life happening again, life stirring."

Jen nods. I can see she is in a not-dissimilar place from the beginning: *How do I do this?* hangs heavily in the air. *Alone?* Only time will tell.

The soup is nice and hot, and we sit down in the bright dining-room. Jen puts placemats down. "New placemats; I bought them yesterday as a birthday present to myself."

Thank god for retail therapy, I think to myself. It's a good sign.

After lunch, we make our way outside. The garden seems to just pull us into it. It's a gorgeous autumn day. The kind everyone hopes Thanksgiving weekend will be like.

"Aren't the leaves amazing this year?" Jen comments. "Did you notice how the leaves changed colour the week Rob was dying?"

Indeed, I had.

"I wonder if more people die in the fall than at any other time of year," Jen ponders. "It just seems so appropriate that in a few weeks we'll be heading into winter, when everything will be dead."

"I don't know if more people die in the fall than in winter, but I do think Rob had an innately amazing sense of timing in everything he did!"

Jen smiles in agreement.

"And remember, Jen," I continue, turning once again to my greatest teacher, the earth, to which my own heart has turned through some long, bleak winters, "Winter isn't dead, Jen. It's fallow. It's when the earth blankets itself with the snows to rest, to gather energy, to renew, ready for the new that rises up in spring. So it is with grief. It feels dead, and your life *has* died. The one you had with Rob.

"I suspect you will need a cocoon of silence, the trees, the back yard, good food, provided by others, of course, to be eaten in small amounts regularly, sleep when your body can sleep, and just literally become like an animal healing, which just does exactly whatever it needs to in its own cave.

"There is so much to assimilate and digest from all this emotionally. It will take a good while, and ahead are moments where the emptiness, the body-ache longing, will overwhelm you, and you need space to *let* it do that. Those waves come with their healing, but only if you can stay diving into them and riding them with breath, trees, silence, music, whatever."

"I just keep thinking," Jen says, with a tone I haven't heard before, of curiosity, something new emerging perhaps, "something over my left shoulder, right here," she gestures to the space next to her left ear, "that something is going to come of this."

I feel my intuition tweaking.

"Tell me more, Jen?" I'm curious.

"The experience I've had in the past fifteen months has been so life altering, I feel I've learned so much about life, hope, love ... all that stuff. I feel like we did this extremely well, and I have no regrets. I feel like everything I could ever have wanted to accomplish to help Rob leave this place I did.

"And although it's awful, and I just feel like I have no idea how I'll do this, I also feel that this experience I had is unique. People keep telling me how unique it is. You and Grace keep telling me how unusual it is the way Rob and I did this. I just keep thinking that there's a story here that needs to be told. And I don't exactly know what that means.

"But I just feel," she continues, "like I can't go back to my normal life and my normal job and just put this whole experience on a shelf. Rob's influence through his experience of *living* with this terminal disease has changed a lot of lives. I know it has. The people that shared our story have told me they have been changed by it. So I just can't get that image out of my head that there is something begging for my attention that needs to be done with this."

Here is Jen's incredible resilience rising up again. This is the moment I know without doubt she's going to make it through this. The new shoots are rising up, and already. It's quite remarkable. The 'something new' is finding her. And she's absolutely right.

I've known this since I started cutting and pasting Jen's e-mails and my responses back and forth into a document. For some instinctive reason, I knew this story wanted telling. I've been plugging away quietly, with no idea about how, when, or if that would ever happen.

But now is not the time. This I know as well. Seeds need to stay in the soil, hidden, to gather strength, lest our minds seize them too early and drag them prematurely into form and visibility. Jen's too raw in her grief. She needs to experience the 'becoming' of the new within her first. But life is finding her. For that I feel a well of gratitude rising up.

"Well, Jen, trust that," I gently offer. "Trust the sense of something. Hold it gently without trying to understand it. It will take shape in its own way at the right time. Now's the time for healing and letting it come into being in its own time. This is the time for rest, for gathering your strength and allowing this 'something' to come into being through the healing."

She nods, agreeing, and we sit in silence, the 'something' in the air, invisible.

We sit in silence for a moment, the garden full with a peaceful stillness. A crow flies over in that moment, right in my sightline.

"I've been to the bank," Jen says with some energy. "Apparently I'm not going to starve. The bank guy is arranging my finances so that I don't need to go back to work until the new year. And he's giving me the OK from a financial perspective to build a fence around the back yard. Nine days before Rob died, he sat in the lift chair we got for him and recited a list of the things I'd need to look after in the house! He said, 'Well, Jen, you're going to need to replace this window, and you should get a new stair runner because you've always hated that green one, and build yourself a fence. Hopefully, there will be enough life insurance money that you can do all that.'

"So, I'm getting the fence figured out, and I'll figure out all the other stuff too. These are all the projects Rob and I had planned to do before he was ill. And I think I'm going to take a trip to Florida with the little kids. My parents are there at their condo, and I think it would be a nice thing to do for the kids. Give them a break."

All the 'new' that is compelling her forward into life. Another gift Rob gave her, naming projects to keep her moving forward, as was their way together. How wise he was. How well he loved her. I marvel too at the wisdom of the instincts, when we give them a chance, to take the driver's seat. Here they are, in action, right in front of me, in the life of someone who is shattered by grief.

A fence. Looking around at her garden, I can feel the open borders that have no boundary into neighbours and a business yard. It feels diffuse, uncontained. Grief needs a strong, safe container. A safe place to allow the rivers of feelings to flow. I've long since learned the inner is the outer, the outer is the inner. We create our spaces around us to reflect our inner lives. Jen's intuitive wisdom is nudging her to create borders around her grieving process. Privacy and solitude. How incredibly wise and life affirming.

"That's great, Jen. I love the fence idea. That's your wise instincts at work. And Rob's gift to you, again. It will give you a safe cocoon, especially in spring, when you'll be out in your garden. And Florida, I can imagine that will be great for the kids. Do you feel ready to be away from your home, where you feel Rob and feel held so strongly? Are you sure about Florida? It's hard to be away from home and in others' lives in grieving. Not to mention Disney World!"

I know from my own and others' grief experiences how very difficult dislocation from home can be, as if the psyche is already so fragile that the loss of familiar surroundings and their grounding can be too much.

"Well, we'll see, but I'm going to do it for the kids. They need something to look forward to."

Jen's mom instincts are guiding her too. I can see the wisdom in this too.

It's time for me to leave. The same sense of the energy leaving, nudging me to end and depart.

"I'll get going, Jen. It's been super to see you and be with you in your garden. I love your home and the Englishness of it, especially the garden. I can see Rob's gift in creating a little 'England' here."

In our farewell hug, I feel the solidness of this process. As shattering as it is, Jen's going to be OK. Life is still finding her. Rob is still with her.

Thursday 21 October 2010
Home Visit from Grace

Jen

GRACE IS COMING TODAY. I haven't seen her since the funeral three weeks ago. We've had some e-mail and phone contact, which has surprised me. It's really easy for me to put my CCAC hat on and realize that once a client dies there is no budgetary allowance for continuing contact with a bereaved caregiver. I know that Grace is extending herself to me personally with this visit and all the contacts we've had since Rob's death. I'm so very grateful. I don't know what I would do without her.

Grace arrives, and I greet her at the door. As she walks in, she turns to me and hugs me warmly, and I immediately burst into tears. I realize this is the first time I've greeted her at the door without then taking her into a room where Rob is, and his absence is starkly present. I offer her coffee, and we head into the living-room. She sits in the chair she always sat in when visiting Rob and me, and I sit where I always sat. Rob's absence knifes through my heart with a fierce stab.

Grace says, "Well, this is a different kind of visit, isn't it? He sure left a big hole." As always, she names things directly and honestly, not shying away from the truth of the situation. Something else I'm grateful for in her. I nod my agreement, feeling that hole yawning into a wide abyss, and I can hardly speak, the tears just welling.

Grace, sensing this, I suspect, moves to easier topics. "How are you sleeping, Jen? How are you eating?" We both orient ourselves to the details of health, now mine, as we did many, many times with Rob's.

"Well, I'm not really sleeping terribly well. The sleeping pills are still a godsend, although I'd love to get off them at some point. I'm eating a little bit now. My skin doesn't hurt as much as it did. I guess I'm all right."

"You're doing it, Jen," Grace says, her strong voice wrapping around me. "You're doing it. Sleep will come. And my professional opinion would be that I don't think you should be coming off those sleeping pills anytime too soon. It's only been three weeks!" She gently reminds me.

It feels like an eternity. Time seems to have stood still.

"What did you think about the funeral, Grace?" I ask her. "I realize I'm really missing the ability to talk to Rob about events. We always debriefed about everything. I've no one to do that with now."

"Oh, Jen, it was beautiful. It was very 'Rob.' The songs were lovely. 'Let It Be' and 'Tears in Heaven.' So Rob."

"Well, he planned the whole thing, you know."

"He gave you a beautiful gift in doing that. It's the same gift he gave you all along. He never denied the inevitable. He never left you to deal with the details. The journey you and Rob took together, this whole journey, it's been incredible to witness, Jen. And what was so clear to me, in that funeral, was how much love you had for one another. How well you had prepared for that moment, how well you had prepared your children ... "

She pauses and adds, "I've learned an incredible amount from you, Jen. I learn something from every person I walk with" — she gestures quotes around 'walk' — "in their journey towards death, but you and Rob have really taught me about love."

It stuns me to hear Grace speak in this way. It touches me deeply and startles me a bit to hear her using language like this and saying she's learned from us. Grace has been a rock I've leaned on over and over. It never occurred to me that anyone could learn anything from us. I've felt so fragile and tenuous so often. What could anyone learn from that?

She must see my look of surprise, because she explains, "Rob and you truly lived this last year. You grabbed hold of every moment that you had and maximized its potential. You accepted this with such grace. You've proven in the past year that you have an incredible amount of strength and wisdom and courage and resilience.

"This will be an incredibly difficult journey, Jen. And I have no doubt that this journey you're about to embark on will be much harder than the one you and Rob have been on together in the past year. But you'll get through this.

"I'll be here, Helen will be here. Your parents will be here. Your children will be here. And Rob will be here. I have no doubt that Rob will help you get through this. You'll be OK, Jen."

"He *is* here, Grace," I tell her. I want her to know this. "He's all around. I feel him all the time. I must sound like a crazy person, but I do. It was such a privilege to be on that journey with him. And although it was so difficult, I wouldn't have traded it for the world. I needed to be with Rob to get him through this. I was with Rob because I was the person to do it, because I *could* do it. I don't believe that life is all pre-determined, but I do believe that there was a reason we came together all those years ago. And I think the reason was so that I could help him die, because he couldn't have done it alone."

I start crying, and Grace hands me a Kleenex box. There are many lying around my house these days.

She suggests, "Let's go for a walk." I realize she's already been here for over an hour. I wonder if she has time. But clearly she does, she's making time, and I'm not going to dissuade her.

We head out of the house into a cold, sunny autumn day. The leaves have all fallen off the trees, and winter is in the air.

We weave our way through the town, and as we're walking a shift happens as I ask Grace about how she's doing. The professional relationship is shifting in the sands of intersecting lives. She tells me for the first time about things in her life that have shaped who she is, her family, and some current griefs. We've become two women sharing our stories of family, grief, love, and life.

Without any conscious planning, we wind up at the end of the road that leads to the cemetery where we interred Rob almost three weeks ago. I haven't been back since then. The day of the interment was rainy and cold. Today, we have brilliant sunshine.

"Do you want to see where Rob's ashes are?" I ask spontaneously, surprising myself.

"I was really hoping we'd get there today, Jen. Yes," she responds.

We walk slowly to the cemetery, and I take her to Rob's spot. It has a temporary marker — we have not yet faced the issue of a headstone.

Although we cremated Rob, he wanted a headstone, so people had somewhere to visit. The stems of the roses that we had put down at the interment are still lying on the ground, now dead. Grass has grown in where the hole was.

Grace says, "Well, what a beautiful little cemetery. Did Rob get to see where he was going to be?"

"No," I reply. "I picked out the spot with Malcolm and Rob's kids and Rob's parents. Well, Malcolm really picked it. So, maybe that was Rob."

"I was the one that got to put the ashes in the ground," I tell Grace. "The hole was covered up when they handed me the urn. I wasn't really sure how deep the hole was going to be. But I managed OK. It seems so strange to be back here. My mind is in a very different place than it was three weeks ago."

Grace begins to tell me about a time her family had to pick out a casket. In her inimitable way, she manages to weave together story after story, leavening them with the black humour that only people in grief or health care can appreciate. Before I know it, I am laughing at the ridiculousness of her real stories about death and caskets and silk pillows and undertakers and the craziness of the death business. I catch myself standing, laughing, at Rob's spot in the cemetery, appreciating more than ever what a gift Grace is. Rob would be laughing too, right along with us.

"It's hitting me, Grace," I realize, "that you are the only person in the world who has the perspective to be able to see my personal life of the past year and a half and my professional life going forward. You carry a really interesting position for me because you have the ability to understand both pieces and talk about both pieces because the personal piece will so shape and lend structure to my professional life, and I think you're probably the only one in my life that I could really explain that to. It gives me hope that maybe I can come back to work somehow without losing touch with everything I've lived."

"Oh, I'm really happy to be that for you, Jen. Back at that 'mother ship' we call work. There's no way this won't shape what you do from this point onward, both personally and professionally." Her words are so reassuring.

We meander back to my house, and Grace leaves. Laughter and tears. Tears and laughter. That's about it. Sharing them together. It helps a little.

Friday 12 November 2010
Sanibel Island, Florida

Jen

MY KIDS AND I are in Florida with my parents. We arrived a few days ago. Next week, we're heading to Disney World. It's been hard to be away from my home, where I can feel Rob all around me. I miss the privacy of my own space and the home we cared for together.

But this vacation has been very good for Jack and Haley. Endless days of swimming and sun seem to have washed away much of their grief. And they've had me focusing on them twenty-four/seven, for the first time in over a year. They seem very glad to have me back, which is perhaps how it feels to them.

Today, I'm sitting on the beach at Sanibel Island, off the south coast of Florida and extending into the Gulf of Mexico. It's world-renowned for its shelling. The beaches are literally knee deep in shells at water's edge. The horizon seems endless as we look out into the salty Gulf.

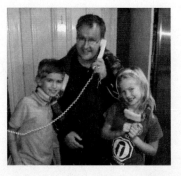

It's an outing we planned so the kids could go shelling and swim in the sea. I've just walked down the beach with Jack and Haley and have come back to deposit their two bags of shells at the feet of the beach chairs where my Mom and Dad are sitting. Jack and Haley have gone down to the water and are playing in the surf. There's a lot of commotion at the beach because someone has just spotted four dolphins — two adults and two babies — not twenty metres from shore.

I've positioned myself on the beach half way between my parents and the kids. I'm sitting on the sand, and there's a beautiful breeze, the sun is shining, its warmth seeping into my skin. I sit quietly as I take in the beautiful surroundings. How I miss Rob. He loved the ocean.

My mind wanders to thinking of the many family holidays and outings that we have spent on beaches. As I sit with my eyes closed, drinking the moment in, I hear Rob's voice inside me saying, "I am the sand."

My mind travels instantly to a time almost exactly a year ago, as we sit in Helen's office, deep in a meditation. She's guiding him to practise changing forms of energy to stay in connection with me. At the end of that meditation, when she asks him what form he had taken, he had become the sand.

I feel the sand supporting me, warming my skin, slipping between my fingers and toes, and I realize he's all around me. I know unequivocally that he is here at this moment with me. I realize that this is not just a diffuse presence in the house because we lived there together and his memories are all around me. He is with me, in me, through me.

And I know now that he's not going anywhere.

He's stayed.

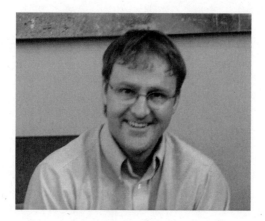

The System and Us

Jen

ROB AND I had been part of the health care system for forty-five years between us when we learned of his diagnosis in August 2009. Much of our
careers we had worked at Parkwood Hospital, a rehabilitation facility directly across the road from the London Regional Cancer Program. Our
drive to the cancer clinic was identical to our long-time daily commute to
work. Being part of the system as both conductors and consumers gave us
a somewhat unique perspective throughout our journey.

Our knowledge of the inner workings of health care — the system's un-
written rules — gave us our first immediate signals about Rob's health
status the day of his diagnosis. The physician's body language when he
walked into the room holding Rob's chart was a stance we both recognized
as one that would accompany very bad news.

After his diagnosis, the acute care unit admitted Rob swiftly to a private
room, listing the reason for admission as "pain control" — code for giving us time to adjust. The unit allowed me to stay overnight, every night,
of Rob's three-day admission, on a small easy chair. Nobody questioned
when I curled up next to Rob in his single hospital bed. The lack of questioning told me how little time he had. Who would dare challenge a wife's
position at her husband's side if he had only a few weeks of life remaining?

It was our knowledge of health care that allowed us to pick up on all these subtle cues. We knew what the norm was for sick but not terminal people. And we recognized how different our treatment was.

At times over the following year, this knowledge served us well. We never wasted any precious time wishing for the impossible, a cure. At other times, the knowledge was harsh, for we never experienced unjustifiable relief.

It was also our awareness of the system's inner workings that permitted us to organize our care so quickly and in a way that worked *for* us. My goal from the very beginning was to have people pay attention to Rob and take an interest in his care. This was my husband, a person. He deserved the very best. He should never need to suffer. He should have the utmost quality of life for the time he had.

I simply could not accept the category of "pancreatic cancer, in treatment room __." I was aware that such a fatal diagnosis would rob him of many privileges. I was never ready to accept the idea that "with this type of cancer there will be pain, suffering, misery, and an imminent death." We had a palliative care physician who thought the same way. I felt management of pain and symptoms to be non-negotiable, and we never tried to negotiate for cure. On many occasions, I pursued the resolution of symptoms that were bothersome, not terrible. My theory was always the same: "If I have only so many days left with Rob, I don't want to waste any of them with a bothersome symptom that we could fix."

I wish I could report that every health care professional pays attention and takes an interest in every patient's care. I believe that this is unfortunately not the case. Physicians often do not have time to review all relevant history. More often than not, they know nothing about the family situation, the level of a patient's "acceptance" or "denial," the presence or absence of support, or the other parties participating. This is no one's fault. It is a result of the system as it has become. Cancer is an ever-more-common diagnosis. Resources are slim and becoming slimmer, and the resources for patients stretched.

When we learned of Rob's diagnosis, I was aware of shortages and of the pressures on many specialists. I knew that there were many people who could be part of our team, not only physicians, and that they could all play a part and pay attention to Rob and round out his care. We never counted on physicians for all our needs. Rob and I were both part of that team, and we knew we could contribute to his care just as skilfully as anyone else.

Reflecting back on our journey, I realize that the impact of the team we assembled was more than that of its individual parts. I believe the level of communication between us all, with Rob and me at the hub of this very complicated wheel, was quite unusual. I wondered openly during the fourteen months of Rob's illness if our level of communication – which I came to rely on and expect — was unusual. I learned that it was. It was perhaps my experience within the system that made me assume I could directly contact team members as an equal.

As the wife and primary caregiver, I knew I had to communicate clearly to advocate for Rob. I needed to speak the language of health care — a tongue we both spoke. We could record symptoms, describe pain, and track side effects. We knew what information the team needed. We became knowledgeable about pancreatic cancer, current research, tools for pain and symptom management, and drugs and their side effects. We knew what to ask the doctors and nurses, what to watch out for.

I still clearly remember the look on Dr Fryer's face on one of her first visits with Rob. She had asked him to describe the pain he was having.

His reply: "I'm having pain in the upper right quadrant, one inch to the right of the sternal notch. The pain is a dull ache, which increases to a sharp stab following ingestion of food. It is precipitated by postural change, specifically by lying flat on my back. It is alleviated by lying on the right side with head elevation. I would rate the pain currently as four out of ten."

Needless to say, this shocked the physician, who recorded Rob's symptoms verbatim on her chart. This is the language of the system. Rob could speak it. It saved us a lot of time and bought us a lot of credibility. It also allowed Rob and me to quickly establish a level of trust with our team. Rob and I became the directors of what was going on. I served as an authority on Rob, and people took my words at face value, trusted my reporting of symptoms, and acted on it immediately. The team valued our contribution and responded accordingly with adjustments to medication, referrals to specialists, or hurrying of timelines.

I do not believe, however, that only insiders can communicate effectively with a health care team. I feel more strongly than ever that this ability involves simply cultivating the skill of good, clear communication.

And who was our team? Rob and I, the palliative care physician, the oncologist, the nurse practitioner, and the spiritual care specialist. At different times, we had also a visiting nurse, a surgeon, chemotherapy nurses, dietitians, endocrinologists, and a case manager. Grace, Helen, and Dr. Fryer were the 'core,' because they all offered me a relationship, not simply a service. I believe we have to have a health care system of individuals who are willing to be intuitive. The concept of "after care" is almost nonexistent in the system but was an essential component of my surviving bereavement.

I also feel that another key to our team's success was the level of intentional communication between all the members. Rob and I had some inkling of the complexities of communication in teams within a complex health care system. Our team spanned at least six organizations:

- London Regional Cancer Program (LRCP)
- Parkwood Hospital, St. Joseph's Health Care London
- Sakura House Residential Hospice
- South West Community Care Access Centre (SWCCAC)
- Tillsonburg Community District Memorial Hospital
- Woodstock General Hospital

A communication link was essential to inform medical players about minute-by-minute changes that can and often do happen with cancer.

Grace very often orchestrated this communication. She would schedule some of her bi-weekly visits for the day prior to our monthly oncologist visits so she could assess Rob thoroughly and e-mail a summary of his current state to the cancer clinic. She was a master of intentional communication and system navigation. She would connect the players who needed connecting, in their own language, and then stay in contact, to keep the focus on Rob and his care.

I often communicated by e-mail, as you can see in this book. It was a thrill and a relief when Grace and Helen each told me I could e-mail or phone them any time.

In addition to keeping the team up to date, e-mail allowed me to convey the complex emotions that went hand in hand with watching my husband succumb to this terrible disease. I had heard of the value of 'journalling' an experience, but for me writing to 'nobody' didn't ever materialize. A one-line e-mail from Grace or Helen checking in and asking "How are you, Jen?" was often all I needed to open the tap for an outpouring of emotions. I don't think I could have traversed this treacherous path without the support I received from them.

There was also a community that held us up and became an essential part of our team as well: family members, friends, neighbours, even strangers. Rob's and my intentional communication through the Rob Update e-mails served to connect us with so many people who held us up through their web of support.

I've thought a lot about the various ingredients that went into Rob's living so well and for so long with such a devastating cancer. The risk in putting any of these ingredients down on paper is that the results may not be reproducible. The unique combination of people, events, timing, and spiritual unknowns led to this remarkable, life-altering experience.

The Authors' Own Stories

Grace

GROWING UP ON A FARM in Ontario, I learned incredible lessons at my mother's knee and felt family support at every stage of my development. This priceless resource has served me well. My mother had trained as a teacher and worked as such very briefly before her marriage. Later she became a stay-at-home Mum whose life revolved around her children. Four of us arrived in her first five years of marriage, and much later, two perimenopausal after-thoughts, with me the 'forever baby.' There followed care to an ageing, demented mother-in-law and being special sister to Eleanor. My mother's whole being was about kindness and compassion to her family and her community.

By the time I was thinking about work, our mother already had two teachers and a secretary among her daughters, so I was the default nurse, the boys of course following Dad into farming. Her friend Mrs. Churchill, who had been a nurse, was a knowledgeable supporter of her persuasive encouragement!

I started in nursing as chief laundress at an Easter Seal Camp for handicapped children near Perth, Ontario. I spent the early 1980s in public health in London and Middlesex County. I worked next at War Memorial Children's Hospital (later Children's Hospital of Western Ontario), managing chronic disease in children with diabetes and cystic fibrosis. My nearly eighteen years in paediatrics in London provided me with a huge repository of experience and great respect for patient-centred, family-focused care delivery.

In 1994, I obtained further credentials, with a master of science in nursing. In 2001, I received certification as a nurse practitioner at the University of Western Ontario. The next year, I started in oncology at the London Regional Cancer Program as an advanced practice nurse in managing fatigue and anaemia — such common complaints for people with cancer. In my eight years there, I was privileged to develop a good rapport with the oncologists and other professionals.

In the summer of 2009, I started as a home-visiting nurse practitioner at the South West Community Care Access Centre, just weeks before I first met Jen and Rob. My patients now are primarily palliative clients, and I see them in their kitchens, living-rooms, and bedrooms. The protection of hospital walls is stripped away, and I need to rely on skills beyond the clinical. My first charge — a family with a dying mother in her eighties — asked me how long I had been in palliative care. I answered truthfully but mentioned my thirty years in nursing.

Cancer care is tough — it's a relentless disease. A lot of sad stories, a lot of loss; at the heart of it, however, people who, despite the psychic and physical pain, rise to another level. My mother's favourite biblical passage was I Corinthians 13, about love conquering everything — and to be witness to this in one's work is beyond understanding, the feelings are so profound.

My own life, with two remarkable young adult children, a home on the farm with all the accoutrements of nature (animal, mineral, and vegetable), and a husband who cares for animals, provides shelter and sustenance for me and meaning in my work.

Helen

I GREW UP in Desborough, in Northamptonshire, in England's Midlands. My parents raised my three sisters and me in the Anglican church, and their own journey through life, grounded always in their faith, formed my profound sense of the sacred in life. They have shown me by example an authentic spiritual journey — a river that flows through a life, giving ground and source to meaning, purpose in chaos, and hope in despair — and that our beliefs should evolve and transform through life. They have taught me too about the heartline of love and prayer and for almost a quarter-century have stayed deeply connected with me despite geographical distance.

My spiritual journey evolved when our theatre group in Toronto met with Henri Nouwen, a contemplative Catholic priest. He wrote about the "broken and lonely heart" — the focus of Jean Vanier's l'Arche communities, with their emphasis on silence and contemplative prayer. He lived in Toronto's l'Arche Daybreak, where I went after leaving the theatre to heal burnout. The residents — young adults with profound mental and physical challenges — embodied presence and called me to authenticity. One young woman, for example, would walk away if she sensed you were not really present; another would not give you her radiant smile if she didn't think you were worth your salt. My months there humbled me.

I went on to the master of divinity program at a Jesuit seminary at the University of Toronto. Some feisty religious sisters there challenged me to listen to the voices of women in theology, which transformed my spiritual life once again. They encouraged me with my thesis on how women's experiences could have enriched language about the Christian deity. To my great surprise, I received the highest marks from all three examiners, one of them the president of the Toronto School of Theology! At that time, my path became about integrating the 'spiritual' with the 'human,' two almost-separate realms in Western society.

Priesthood was out for me — I hadn't vowed to obey my husband, and I certainly wasn't going to vow to obey a bishop! — so I became a chaplain. I worked at St. Michael's and Sunnybrook Health Sciences Centre in Toronto, in trauma intensive care and cardiac intensive care. This immersion into human suffering was life altering. I would see teens dying from car accidents — and comforting their parents. Or parents who were dying — and aiding their spouses and children. In the depths of the night I was called in to baptize newborns who were not making it into life and to support their families. One day I received eleven pages to eleven deaths in a row. I had to grapple with the effects of suffering on our human existence in very concrete ways and ask what on earth spirituality had to do with it all. Death and suffering became my teachers and have taught me over the years how to truly embrace life and really live.

I had married and given birth to two children when we moved out of Toronto to London, Ontario. I began working part time at the London Regional Cancer Program. Balancing a professional life with a family posed a profoundly difficult challenge. I felt an enormous sense of failure at not being a supermom. Two rounds of post-partum depression and distance from my family pushed me into my own descent into darkness.

From the crucible of this descent, I made the very painful decision to end my marriage of ten years and became a single parent. I gave up half the time with my children for their and their father's sake. I was living into our new life and grieving in the gaping hole when they were away. This 'black hole' became my spiritual practice. My parents' grounding turned me towards an innate trust in 'something.' I discovered I too still had a trust 'in life' and that at the heart of life flows a river of wisdom that guides us through the darkness.

During my hard times, I leaned on some extraordinary sources of support. The land of Hawaii has the most extraordinary healing offerings, and there I recovered from the pain of the divorce. Back in London, local native friends — Asayenes, Kilder Clan (Dan Smoke) and Asayenes Kwe, Bear Clan (Mary Lou Smoke) — gave me the teachings of their people with huge love and generosity. Our full moon ceremonies were a monthly medicine seeping into my bones; the earth is indeed a mother and teacher and what a gift that has been to my children and me and the many other people who over the years have gathered around the sacred fire to offer their struggles and prayers.

My Jungian analyst, Douglas Cann, proved a profoundly wise guide during my deep descent and taught me that our dreams support and nourish us wisely. Pretty much all that I could offer to Jen and Rob came from the unshakeable trust-in-life that I could touch into during my sessions with Douglas. Carl Jung recognized death and resurrection as an archetypal force at the centre of the human psyche and human experience and that it shapes our dreams. To find its meaning for us, we must dive into our suffering and grapple, as Jacob did with the Angel of God, for the 'blessing,' or the gold, from the experience.

Whom one prays to can become quite irrelevant when one is facing death, as Jen and Rob discovered. The real journey of faith then begins in prayer, it seems to me, when one searches, wrestles, weeps, struggles, and crawls through the experience, crying out, "I will not give up, there has to be a way through this." This is the reality that Jen and Rob's story unfolds. It is a journey of the most heartbreaking 'faith' and the most hope-filling encounter with 'life' in its loving wisdom or grace. Stripped bare by tragedy, we begin the journey into the heart of life in utter darkness of heart and mind. What we discover is deeply personal, and one person's story can provide only hope for another, not an answer, because there is none, only a way. This way we can discover only moment by moment, breadcrumb by breadcrumb, as we trek through the forest of life.

Liz White, founder of the Psychodrama Institute in Canada, a true wisewoman elder, has guided me through the griefs and celebrations of each stage in my journey. Lucinda Vardey opened me to the notion of the divine feminine, pulled me under her wing during my seminary days, and taught me, in her spiritual life retreats, to teach experiential process from the gestalt basis.

Looking at and listening to my own soul pain through dreams, dialogue, meditation, journalling, and all manner of inwardly nourishing activities, plus having the lifeline of skilled, healing relationships, allowed me to survive my descent. I'm not sure we can get through such a journey intact without the loving and wise guide who has one foot in 'trust-in-life' when we do not. Through all these relationships, I have forged my own integrative approach to life and living. It has been a long and slow journey of healing.

We providers of clinical interfaith spiritual care have to be authentic but also spiritually 'multilingual,' and I respect each person's perspective and paradigm deeply. The word 'god' is not often in my personal vocabulary; for me, there is no longer any separation between 'god' and anything else, just the all-encompassing force we call 'life' in all its transcendent experiences and its great, vast, and wise depths.

In the London Regional Cancer Program, I found that this terrible disease could be a potent catalyst for transformation, and all of this prepared me for my remarkable journey with Jen and Rob. When Grace called me in August 2009 to meet with them, I was in the midst of this reintegration of my life and emerging into a surprising sense of wholeness. I had listened to many courageous individuals who had picked their way through the shattering impact of cancer and discovered their unique and unbreakable wholeness within it. I thus found I was able to meet Jen and Rob with my own bone-deep discovery that in the depths of our psyche and life lies a wisdom that is compassionate, supportive, nurturing, and always weaving life into the situations that seem to shatter us. I came to a profound trust in the process that can happen in the depths of despair. This was the only gift I had to offer them, and I hoped very much that it might be enough.

Jen

IT FEELS STRANGE to write about myself when most of the preceding pages have been about my life with Rob. I will endeavour to fill a few gaps.

I grew up in the country on a sixty-acre property in Flamboro, Ontario, near Hamilton. It was a small farm, and my parents, John and Maureen Vickers, rented out the 'back forty' to a neighbouring farmer. As a child, I wished I lived in town, closer to friends and fun, but, looking back, I see an idyllic place for my parents to raise my brother, John, and me. We grew up as 'Jenny and Johnny,' got along pretty well, and still do. He owns a foundry in a small Ontario town, and reminds me more and more of our Dad.

Our parents were both professionals with university degrees, which was somewhat unusual among our friends and acquaintances. They always told us we were smart and could do whatever we wanted to; I knew John and I would go to university and find satisfying work and financial independence. When we were kids, our mechanical-engineer Dad ran a small engineering company designing air-pollution control systems for the steel industry in Hamilton and later was vice-president of a successful foundry. Mom has a degree in nursing and, when we were young, co-ordinated home care in the community for people with various types of illnesses. She later became a director at Parkwood Hospital in London, where both Rob and I had also worked.

When I was nine, our (maternal) Grandma Rita was diagnosed with terminal cancer at Tillsonburg Hospital (the same!). I listened intently to many hushed conversations, especially a phone chat Mom had in our kitchen. When I asked her why she was crying, she told me, "Grandma has cancer." When I asked her what the doctors would do, she replied, "Nothing, Jenny. There's nothing they can do. She will die, and we will try and make sure she's comfortable."

Grandma stayed a few days in hospital, and then her family took her home — highly unusual back in the 1980s. The three daughters essentially moved in to look after her, their husbands maintaining home and children. I clearly remember visiting her, sick but in her own bed, in the three weeks before she died. She passed away peacefully in her own bed, in the tender care of her family. To me growing up, this way of dying seemed as natural as the sky is blue.

Just as my brother followed in Dad's footsteps, I followed in Mom's. I studied biology at the University of Western Ontario in London. My very first job was as a rehabilitation therapist at Parkwood Hospital in the Acquired Brain Injury Program, and I later took on more significant clinical roles. After a recruitment firm approached me, I interviewed successfully for project manager in London at the South West Community Care Access Centre, where I received promotions over the years — and tremendous support when I left to look after Rob in August 2009. I have since returned to work there, and some of my projects involve palliative and end-of-life care and looking at how we can improve the experience for patients and families.

And, above all, I am mother to Haley and Jack and stepmother to Jessica and Ben — my most rewarding and challenging roles. In Rob's illness and death, we have experienced something I wouldn't wish on any young person. And, as you saw above, Rob and I, our families, and our team worked together to shepherd our dear children through the experience. We talked and still talk very openly about Rob and about everything we've gone through together. I'm so proud and glad to have had the extraordinary opportunity to witness it all and, with my fellow authors, to share it with you.

Acknowledgments

Grace

THIS ACCOUNTING OF THE LIVES and the love of Jen and Rob has been a privilege of witness for me. They invited me to be their "system navigator," confidante, and nurse practitioner, and I am very grateful to them. I am thankful that the leadership at the South West Community Care Access Centre, where I had just started, entrusted me to provide care to this special couple. My eight years of experience at the London Regional Cancer Centre and the trusting relationships that I forged there helped me to bridge the community and the Cancer Centre environs for Jen and Rob. I am grateful to Dr. Karen Fryer for her commitment to collaborative care, which allowed for my full engagement in this man's care. I feel gratitude for my thirty-five years in nursing roles and for my opportunities for advanced education, which have contributed to my way of being as a nurse practitioner in this world of community palliative care.

This book began as a reflection of communications between formal and informal care providers and has reached this present state with the encouragement of many people: Judy Maddren, who gave us our first objective review; Judy's husband, Tim Elliott, who connected us with John Parry, our very sensitive editor and publisher; my sister Margaret McDowell, who put us in touch with her friend Maxine Trottier, a 'real' writer, whose guidance, support, and editorial suggestions took us yet another step towards publication.

Lastly, I am grateful to Jen and Helen for their creative writing, which has shaped this narrative beautifully as a reflection of the love and work that carried Rob and Jen through their journey. May those who bear witness to that in their reading take heart.

Helen

I HAVE LEARNED from the many courageous women and men in history that we never accomplish anything without standing on a long line of shoulders, visible and invisible, paving the way and guiding us. For the First Nations people of this land, Turtle Island, this includes our ancestors and the 'life-support system' we call the earth, and this reality has become very true for me. There have been many helpers along the way to the birthing of this book and my role in co-writing it.

Without my parents, Joyce and Graham Butlin, and their unconditional love, listening ears, and hours of dialogue from our diverging and intersecting points of view, my spiritual journey would not have taken place in the way it did. They are truly my elders-in-life and stand behind the woman who helped pen these pages.

My spiritual teachers and companions through my struggles have been integral to this process: Douglas Cann, Dan and Mary Lou Smoke, Lucinda Vardey and her husband, John Dalla Costa, and Liz White, and, behind them, the insights and wisdom of Carl Jung. They have interwoven with all that happened in the alchemy of this journey with Jen and Rob and their children.

I thank my leaders at the London Regional Cancer Program, who have supported me in a role that has been difficult to integrate into the medical system. They provided the container for my role that allowed this journey to happen as it did. They trusted my highly intuitive, non-linear way of doing things and have allowed a unique service to develop. Without their support for me and for spiritual care within the cancer program, through much adversity, this story would not have happened.

The village of support around me consists of my dearest and trusted friends — Sheilagh Ashworth, Stacey Bothwell, Deborah Graham, Mary-Bee Haworth, Cathy Jenniskens, Kris McNab, Tina Plat-Dekoter, and Victory. They have formed the fabric of my own support system for me and my children to sustain the emotional rigours of walking with people who are suffering, and they have all walked with me personally through the emotional impact of witnessing the profound soul pain of this journey. I must especially acknowledge Carol Dunphy and Elizabeth Pickett, who have been my greatest teachers in honouring the rawness of another person's soul pain without seeking the band-aid of hope before it is genuinely born from the others' lived experience. Their own presence in my heart helped me to stay silent many times with Jen and Rob when I would have been tempted to offer inadequate and meaningless words.

I thank my children for teaching me to embrace my humanity and stop fighting or pretending it shouldn't exist and for their remarkable capacity to just be themselves and embrace life wholeheartedly. Also, my gratitude for their willingness to entertain themselves as I spent hours and hours crafting and editing the earliest versions of this book while not always being the best mother and for their forgiving me anyway!

Kasia D'Alassandro deserves special mention for being one of the 'invisible gifts' that showed up at just the right moment. Kasia devoted hours to correcting our punctuation, spelling, and grammar to make the text presentable for the first draft that we sent to Judy Maddren. Judy gave us the courage to believe this was a story that could make its way into the lives of people who may value it as 'bread' for their journey. And thanks to Judy as well for linking us to John Parry, this book's humble, exquisitely sensitive editor and publisher. His keen insight into the heart of the story and his intuitive grasp of the essence of Rob, which is present on every page, made him the perfect person to assist with its birth into a book.

Finally, I honour Jen and Grace deeply for the interweaving of our professional lives and this deeply connecting journey together and then for the process of creating this book together. It has been a remarkable collaboration of 'best practice' professionally, of the strength of women's friendships through struggle, and of the laughter that rises up between us like an irrepressible force of strength, even in the most painful of times. Thanks for the many cups of tea, glasses of wine, shared meals, and incredible sharing of our lives as professionals and as women that make this story so alive and rich.

Without Rob's being who he was, none of this story would be written. A deep bow of respect to a man who faced death with true wisdom and the most powerful love for his beloved Jen and their children. He revealed to me the reality of love that truly can transcend the grave, and it has changed my life. I thank him.

Jen

CONTRARY TO WHAT many people may believe once they read this book, there are moments these days when I feel like the luckiest woman in the world. I have been the recipient of countless acts of human kindness and generosity since the time of Rob's cancer diagnosis. I wish I could thank every individual who has extended his or her hand to me over the past few years, but that would render the acknowledgments longer than the book itself.

I thank my parents, John and Maureen Vickers, and my brother, John, who provided me the upbringing I needed to live through the past few years, the practical support to manage through the tough times, and the unwavering love and support to Rob and me and our family. I thank also Rob's parents, Brian and Mildred Fazakerley, who supported Rob and his family across the ocean throughout his twenty-three years in Canada and who provided so much support and love to Rob and me and our children during his illness. I thank as well Rob's brothers and their wives, Andrew and Lorraine, Malcolm and Caroline, Howard and Lynn, who all made it to Canada to spend cherished time with Rob before he died.

My children and stepchildren, Haley, Jack, Jessica, and Ben, have endured much and have all survived and thrived. I am so proud of all of them. More than anything, they have provided me with a reason to keep going, a reason to continue to keep Rob's memory alive. They each embody a piece of Rob that I see every day and treasure. My heartfelt thanks to each of them.

I have an amazing group of friends that I refer to as 'The Parkwood

Girls.' They have been my friends and Rob's, and they form the most thoughtful and practical group of supporters, cheerleaders, encouragers, and shoulders to lean and cry on. They provided my family and me with groceries, fund-raisers, hand-me-downs for kids, scrapbooks of cards, girls' weekends away, and much, much more. They continue to be there whenever I need them. I thank Lana Rossi, Monique Crites, Julie Hughes, Lisa McCorquodale, Kelly Williston-Wardell, Anne-Marie Kap, and Jill Bowen-Good. I couldn't have asked for more from these women. Also my gratitude to everyone at Parkwood Hospital, particularly Rob's colleagues, who kept him engaged in his beloved place of work. Special thanks to Anna Kras-Dupuis (formerly Anna Bluvol) for all of her support. I know that Rob's memory lives on in the walls of Parkwood and in the many stories that are shared about him.

A particular word of thanks to my very dearest friend, Julia Upton. As a physician, Julia was my go-to expert for the complexities that Rob and I faced in the world of cancer, and she was also my closest confidante and oldest friend. It was Julia's words and unwavering belief in my strength that kept me going on many a difficult night. She sat next to me at Rob's funeral and handed me Kleenex and told me, as only a friend of over twenty years could, that she knew I would get through it all. And I have.

My employer, the South West Community Care Access Centre, supported me in my leaving my job to be where I needed to be when Rob was ill and always let me know I would have a job to come back to. I can hardly express my gratitude for the constant support and encouragement. I would like to thank particularly Donna Ladouceur, for her sensitive and steadfast kindness and solicitude throughout Rob's illness and her support in my return to work.

A remarkable team looked after Rob throughout his illness, and its remarkable members deserve my especial gratitude. In particular, the exceptional clinical skills that Dr. Karen Fryer called on were complemented by her gentle, respectful, kind manner, and she provided my dear husband with incredible palliative and end-of-life care. We were so lucky to have found her.

Without Helen and Grace, there would be no book. The first six months I spent as a widow, they cocooned me, and they each helped me in their own unique way. We have evolved from members of a care team, to co-authors, to dear friends. We have enjoyed holidays together, presented at conferences together, and shared many a meal with each other and each other's families. I am so blessed to have them in my life.

It was Helen's exceptional writing skills that allowed us to capture many of the written 'stories' within the book. We spent hours and hours at her house, with her typing furiously on her computer while I recounted memories of my days with Rob that were essential to fill in the blanks between the correspondence e-mails. She would tease out the emotion attached to the facts and caught them beautifully. I thank her.

Grace was responsible for my physical recovery from the harrows of grief, and a tremendous support as I re-entered the working world. She and I have evolved into work colleagues now as well as friends, and for that I am truly grateful. She often provides me with a much-needed lunch or coffee break, or often just a quick e-mail to check in, and somehow always encourages me to stop and breathe. My thanks to her.

I thank the people in my life who have supported me and encouraged me to carry on, to smile, and to laugh. My gratitude goes to them for showing me that life is still out there and that I don't have to 'go it alone.'

And finally, Rob. It was an honour and a privilege to be his partner. How to put into words how deeply and completely I love him and always will, no matter what my future brings. He has made such a difference in so many lives, and I hope that process continues through the words in this book. I know it will. Even in his death, he is carving out a future for me that is full, and happy, and meaningful. He was and is amazing. And I thank him, from the bottom of my very full heart.

So What Is It Like Now?

Jen

"DO YOU FEEL ROB'S PRESENCE?"

My friends ask me questions such as this quite often. Answering them puts me out on a bit of a limb. There are a lot of notions about what should happen when a loved one dies. At different points in my life, I have had many ideas on the subject. I suppose even my limited exposure to religious beliefs about what happens after we die has fed into many of my thoughts: angels, heaven, purgatory, reincarnation, and so forth.

But my current beliefs have emerged from my personal experience of the year of Rob's illness and the time since he died.

About a week after Rob's diagnosis with cancer, we went for a walk down the road in front of our house. It was a beautiful day in August, with the sun shining on the colourful leaves that were just beginning to change, and my world falling to pieces before my eyes. As we were walking — slowly, because Rob was in such pain — he said to me, "I'll always be with you, Jen. I'll be right there with you wherever you are, whispering in your ear. All you'll have to do is listen. I'll never leave you." This was before we met Helen and heard about the heartline, before we started meditating together to strengthen the bonds between us. This was Rob's core belief, and it is mine.

I believe that Rob is still very much with me. I feel his presence always. At times, I feel him in a very physical, sensorial way. I will 'hear' him saying something funny in his charming Liverpool accent, or I will sense him standing next to me as I prepare a meal in the kitchen. Sometimes, I will 'feel' him lay his hand on my shoulder when I am sad. But all these sensorial feelings pale in comparison to the energetic, emotional bond that I still feel with him.

The best way I can think to describe it is to say that I still feel as loved by Rob today as I did when he was alive. To describe this feeling is almost impossible, because, at least in my personal experience before now, I have felt loved only by other living people. But the love that I continue to feel from Rob extends to a very different place. It is an energy, or a currency, that feels infused into everything I do. I feel that I am better able to manage the challenges in my life, and experience its joys, because I know Rob is with me, and he loves me. This feeling is no different now from when he was alive and I knew that he loved me. It's impossible to explain to someone who hasn't had the experience. And, to be honest, I have no idea if other people have this experience. I know only what this is like for me.

At first, it was like wisps of him in and out. And they were so crushed under the absence of him and my sadness. I felt so flat, I was there, but I felt awful, empty. I'd have these moments and laugh at something and then remember he wasn't there. The feeling of 'him' was fleeting, as if he was still 'here' standing near me.

Things are different now. It feels like he's more 'in me' and 'through me,' rather than 'beside me.' The feeling I used to have when he was beside me was that he could just as quickly not be beside me. If I felt like I ever really needed to feel him, he would almost always deliver something, a dream or a feeling.

Now it's *through* me. I feel that Rob is solidly with me, helping me live my life in partnership with me as he did when he was physically present. It's as if he's figured out how to be in my life even though he is gone. I feel that I am in a place where he is with me always in the decisions and actions that I take. There's a plan evolving, and we're working on it together.

I'm sure it would be easy to explain away this feeling as a side effect of grief. Truly, if I had read in 2005 of a new widow describing an energetic, loving relationship with her dead husband, I would have suggested she seek psychiatric help. Hence the limb I feel that this puts me on. But I don't believe this is an illness, or a poor coping strategy. I believe the continuing bond I feel with Rob is a result of the strong love we had between us when he was alive, and I believe that bond is stronger than death.

Rob and I often remarked that we must have known each other before in "some other life" because of the ease of conversation and immediate closeness and comfort we had around each other. I often wonder now if this may really be the case. I suppose I'll never know. I do know that I was meant to meet Rob when I did. I know that I needed to come into his life so I could help him in his death — of that I am absolutely sure.

I know that if Rob could have spared me the pain that I have endured in watching him succumb to this disease and slip away, he would have. He would have done anything to protect me, all of us, from this. I also know that if I could have gazed into a crystal ball when we fell in love, and had been able to see this in my future, I wouldn't have changed a thing. I wouldn't have traded in those six wonderful years with him for anything, even if I had known it would end like this.

On occasion, in the time leading up to Rob's death and afterwards, there were people who commented to me that I didn't deserve this. This comment always upset me greatly. Of course, no one deserves to become a widow when they are thirty-six, but I always felt that this comment somehow minimized or eliminated the tender, beautiful, unexpected gifts that come with death.

I can't imagine doing anything for someone that is a more strong expression of love towards them than helping them die. I feel that the level of connection that formed between Rob and me in the year leading up to his death was a tremendous gift that we gave one another, and I'm not sure that it would have formed in different circumstances.

I have no doubt that if we had had the opportunity to grow old together, we would have eventually come to feel the connection that developed in the last year of his life, but I think it might have been more diffuse. This is not to say that I wouldn't do anything to have Rob back. I would do anything to be able to hug him just one more time, or hear his laugh, or feel the warmth of him next to me in bed at night, but that is not going to happen. The connection between us is continuing, and I have no reason to think it will not keep doing so.

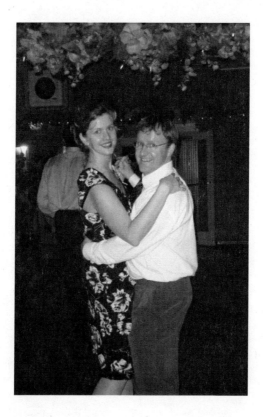

Rob and I had a wonderful six years together.
It was an honour and a privilege to be his partner
and walk this journey with him.

— Jen

Just Stay ... was
designed by *Anne Vellone* of
vellone design & communications
in the beautiful summer of 2012 in
Toronto. 1000 copies were printed &
bound by *Advertek*, using elegant
and classic Berkeley Oldstyle
and Frutiger typefaces.

vellone**design**

www.vellonedesign.com